Celebrating Grandmothers

Grandmothers talk about their lives

Ann Richardson

New Generation **Publishing**

For
James and Owen

Contents

Preface _____ 9

Chapter 1: The Joy of Grandmothers _____15

Chapter 2: Becoming a Grandmother ____19

Being told about the pregnancy _____ 19
    Hearing the news _____ 19
    First thoughts _____ 23

Involvement in the pregnancy _____ 25
    Levels of involvement _____ 25
    Giving advice _____ 28

The birth _____ 30
    Helping out _____ 30
    Seeing the baby for the first time _____ 34

The first weeks _____ 36
    Helping the new mother _____ 36
    Early signs of problems _____ 38

Chapter 3: Doing Things Together _____41

Levels of involvement _____ 41
    Regular arrangements _____ 41
    Living together _____ 44
    Distant grandchildren _____ 46

Activities with grandchildren _____ 50
    Babies and toddlers _____ 50
    Young grandchildren _____ 51
    Older grandchildren _____ 55
    Grown-up grandchildren _____ 58

Coping with lots of grandchildren _____ 59

Family get-togethers _____ 61

Holidays together _____ 64

Keeping in touch _____ 66

Chapter 4: The Emotional Side _____ 70

Love and its expression _____ 70
   Watching them grow _____ 75
   Feeling connected _____ 77
   Physical contact _____ 78
   Talking about the grandchildren _____ 82
   Worrying _____ 86
   Happy memories _____ 92

Favourites and not so favourites _____ 95

Those with little or no access to their grandchildren 99

Individual grandchildren _____ 103

Chapter 5: Views on Child-Rearing _____ 108

Parental approval _____ 108

Disagreements on child-rearing _____ 109
   Material things _____ 110
   The use of time _____ 110
   Other issues _____ 112
   Larger problems _____ 114

Offering advice _____ 115
   Daughters and daughters-in-law _____ 119
   Changing views about managing children _____ 121

Looking after the grandchildren _____ 123
   Spoiling _____ 126
   Involvement in discipline _____ 127

Helping with problems _____ 131
    Issues or problems at home _____ 132
    Understanding themselves _____ 133
    Wider questions _____ 136

Chapter 6: The Image and Role of
Grandmothers_____137

The image of grandmothers _____ 137
    Own grandmothers _____ 140
    Own mothers as grandmothers and mothers ___ 144

Kinds of grandmother _____ 147
    Providing childcare or not _____ 147

The many aims of grandmothers _____ 152
    Supporting the parents _____ 152
    Helping the grandchildren _____ 154
    Fostering a sense of family _____ 157
    Long-term relationships _____ 159
    Financial involvement _____ 163

Chapter 7: The Impact on Other
Relationships_____166

The son-in-law or daughter-in law (or partner) ___ 166
    The good stories _____ 166
    Strained relationships _____ 168
    Absent partners _____ 172

The son or daughter with the grandchildren _____ 174

The other grandmother(s) _____ 179

Other children _____ 184

Grandfathers and their role _____ 187
    Absent grandfathers _____ 191

Chapter 8: Looking Back and Looking Forward _____ 194

Looking back on parenthood _____ 194
*The regrets*_____ 194
*Making amends*_____ 196
*Proud mothers*_____ 198
*Easier to be a grandmother than a mother*_____ 200

Being part of a line _____ 203
*Seeing a family resemblance*_____ 203
Family traditions _____ 206

Looking forward_____ 210
Hopes for the future _____ 210
*Concerns for the future*_____ 214
Being a burden _____ 218
*The fragility of life*_____ 222

Chapter 9: Reflections on Being A Grandmother _____ 225

Finding the right balance _____ 225
Keeping the right distance _____ 225
Having their own life _____ 226
Moving to be near the family _____ 230

The status of grandmothers _____ 235
Feeling valued _____ 235
Being a matriarch _____ 240
Wisdom _____ 244

Missing out on the pleasures _____ 247

End thoughts_____ 249

Preface

This is a book about the lives and views of grandmothers, as told by grandmothers themselves. So, you might ask, who wants to read about a lot of wrinkled old ladies? Well, for a start, wrinkled old ladies themselves, who tend to be largely ignored in books and the media. Plus the not-so-wrinkled, since some women become grandmothers in their forties or even earlier and some, who are not yet grandmothers, have an interest in understanding the stage of life they will be reaching soon. Not to mention the occasional person who might like to know what that quiet woman in the corner seat is thinking about.

The main reason I wanted to write this book is because I have found being a grandmother fascinating. Not just fascinating, but completely and surprisingly so. I had no idea of the significance it would have in my life. My own grandmothers were moderately absent – one because she lived a long distance away and we saw her very infrequently and the other because she had only a very limited interest in her grandchildren. My children, also, had little involvement with their grandmothers – my husband's mother had died before they were born and my mother was a long way away and more engaged in her career. So, for me, there was no model for this stage in my life and certainly no very positive one.

Yet from the moment of birth of my first grandson, I felt immensely involved. I was keen to watch him – and the second, his cousin, who came along three years later – develop. I felt they were both very much part of my life and my planning. I did not want to go away for too long, because I wanted to keep up with changes in their lives. I not only adored them and the fun I had with them, but I liked the 'me' that I became with them.

I realised that it was much easier to be a granny than a mother and felt I was doing better at it. I probably became a bore to family and friends, talking about them and the funny things they said, although no one has ever told me so.

Yes, being a grandmother added a whole new layer to my life. But this was not solely due to the new members of the family to love and to worry about. There were also new territories to be negotiated, like when and how to offer advice to the parents without getting their backs up. As I took on occasional childcare, I had to remember both the practical and the more complex emotional sides of looking after them. And perhaps most surprising of all, I had to come to terms with a very new image of myself as a grandmother – the older generation, with all that this implies.

It seemed such an obvious focus for a book that I was surprised it had not been done before, at least in this way. I checked it out and found the occasional book by an individual grandmother and a considerable number of books offering advice, with various titles around the theme of how to be a good granny. Indeed, I found one enticingly subtitled 'how to be a bad grandmother'. But I didn't want to give advice – I wanted to show how it felt from the inside. Of course, there may be much to be learned from what these grandmothers have to say and different readers may take different messages from their thoughts. But my focus was on letting them talk about their lives.

This book is not about the grandchildren, no matter how many clever things they say or do. Evidently, some grandchildren, when they learned of this project, automatically assumed that such a book would be about them – as one teenage granddaughter asked 'What do they want to know about *me*?' The grandmothers themselves, however, had no difficulty understanding that they – and their emotions – were the focus of attention, although some were keen to talk about their grandchildren as well.

As I was writing this book, one friend asked if I had a thesis – was there a particular point that I was trying to make, using the interviews to prove it? The answer is a resounding no. It was never my intention to prove anything, aside from the multiplicity of perspectives and experiences of grandmothers in different circumstances. I did not know what I would find when I set out, and can only say that I was delighted with the varied nature of the responses.

One question was how to find my grandmothers. When I first told friends that I was planning this book and looking for people to interview, more often than not if they were grandmothers themselves, they would say cheerfully 'You could interview me'. But it is unprofessional to interview anyone you know, so I had to decline. I began by approaching people in a park and shopping centre and found two or three in this way. But I then discovered that while I could not interview my friends, I could interview *their* friends. So I asked neighbours about their friends and friends about their friends and neighbours. I asked people I knew from various activities I do and, on occasion, local shopkeepers. One woman phoned me and asked to take part without my ever knowing how she heard of the project. As I was very concerned to talk to people with a range of backgrounds, I always talked briefly to the women on the phone to learn something about them prior to the interview. This also, of course, gave them a chance to ask more about the planned book.

What can be said is that these grandmothers come in all shapes and sizes. Some are old, some are surprisingly young, some elegant and some struggling. In the end, we spoke to 27 grandmothers. All but one lived in

London (the exception was interviewed on a visit to London), but they lived in all corners of this diverse city – East, West, North and South London. We interviewed one living in Kensington (for those not familiar with London, this is one of the richest areas) and several in Tower Hamlets (one of the poorest). The majority were born in the UK – indeed, many of these were born in London itself – but because London is a very cosmopolitan place, a considerable number also came from elsewhere. Their countries of origin included, in no particular order, Australia, France, Pakistan, Iran, Nigeria, Sweden, Zimbabwe, Egypt and Barbados. They also spanned the major religions: Christian, Jewish, Muslim, Hindu.

The ages of those we interviewed ranged from 46 to 88, but many had first become grandmothers long before – the youngest at age 36. They had worked in a myriad of occupations, including a former teacher, writer, postwoman, civil servant, child-minder, finance director, singer, and cleaner, to name some examples. A few had been housewives all their lives. Some continued to work. Some had only one grandchild, while some had grandchildren in high numbers, the jackpot going to a woman with eleven. The ages of the grandchildren ranged from a few months to age 29. Three were great-grandmothers and a couple of others had great-grandchildren on the way.

This is not, of course, a 'representative' sample, nor was it meant to be. There are probably surveys that can tell you the proportion of grandmothers who look after their grandchildren full-time or see their grandchild less than once a month. This was never the purpose of this book. Instead, it was intended to provide a sense of the texture of grandmothers' lives – the complexities of their feelings and the diversity of their experiences. The same project, undertaken at another time or by another person, would interview 27 completely different people. Their individual stories and the way they expressed themselves would clearly not be identical, but I suspect the general picture would be very much the same.

Interviews of the kind used for this book are very open and fluid – there is no formal questionnaire and no effort to put people's responses into pre-set boxes. Instead, there is a rough 'topic guide', developed in advance, that helps the interviewer to remember the range of issues to be covered. But essentially, each interview is a conversation and each invariably goes in a slightly different direction. Indeed, not every person is even asked every question. Sometimes, time runs out. A person might have a particularly compelling story to tell. Sometimes, we think of an interesting line of questioning only after the first interviews have taken place.

All interviews were recorded and transcribed verbatim, that is word for word. It is this process that allowed me to use the interviews thoroughly. I read them over very carefully many times and then edited down the contributions so they were manageable to read. I made the decision to correct the English of those who were not native English speakers or who did not always speak grammatically, as I feel it gives people more dignity to be presented in this way. In all other ways, these are the words of the grandmothers themselves and many different voices can be heard.

Because the interviews were very intimate and open discussions, some grandmothers shared thoughts that they would not want traced back to them, particularly about relationships within their family. This caused me a dilemma in how to use the contributions without hurting the person – or their family – in any way. I had always said that no real names would be used. In the end, I decided not even to use pseudonyms because those with very individual and recognisable stories might be traced through. Very occasionally, I have mildly changed certain details so that no one could be fully identified by family or friends. This may be annoying to the reader, who might like to note the thoughts of individual women, but it is a necessary protection to the grandmothers themselves who spoke with such honesty about their lives.

I am, of course, enormously grateful to my interviewer, Paul Vallance, who carried out the discussions with great sensitivity and skill. He had to respond quickly and thoughtfully to very different individuals and circumstances. A number of those interviewed commented subsequently on how pleasurable it was to reflect on the issues raised, some of which they had not directly thought about before. I am also grateful to my two transcribers, who had to listen to the discussions through the occasional veil of barking dogs, whirring dishwashers, local car alarms and the like, which seem be much more of a distraction in a recording than in real life. I must also thank highly all the friends, acquaintances and neighbours who allowed me to pester them for the names and contact details of grandmothers they knew.

And most of all, I give tremendous thanks to all the grandmothers in this book, who dug deeply both into their memories and into their innermost thoughts about their current circumstances to recount a range of complex – often happy, but sometimes painful – experiences. The book could not, needless to say, have been written without them.

Chapter 1
The Joy of Grandmothers

Television documentaries often begin with short clips from the main body of the programme, serving as a 'taster' for what is to come. In this short introduction, a few women talk about being a grandmother, again to serve as a taster for the main text. These are not repeated anywhere else, however.

First, there is the fact that the joy of being a grandmother comes as a complete surprise:

> For years and years my friends used to come up to me and say, with great enthusiasm 'I'm a granny!' And I would think, well, *you* haven't done anything. How can you be so excited, as if you've achieved something? You're only a granny – it's not as though you've produced the baby. Producing the baby is the great thing. So I ignored all my friends, I wasn't interested in their grandchildren at all.
>
> And then I had my own grandchildren and I just fell in love with them – each one is more wonderful and more perfect and more of a marvel than the one before. I've got more involved in looking at them and observing them as time has gone.
>
> *grandmother of five*

Second, there is the love and involvement with so many new people as a result:

> Being a grandmother is such a different stage of life. It's very maturing in a way – and it's also a tremendous challenge. There is this beautiful

love relationship unencumbered by excessive responsibility. And you see all the family strands playing through. It's like a form of weaving, the fabric of families coming together and you start to write another story together – I find that so moving. Suddenly we're making this new fabric. It is quite amazing – it's wonderful, very enriching – this other stage of life.

grandmother of three

Being a grandmother – and sometimes also a great-grandmother – becomes central to a woman's life:

I've been a grandparent for 30 years now, so it's hard to think of myself as not being one. You have this whole bunch of people who you want to keep connections with. All my life, in a way, has been centred around the family. Emotionally, they take up an awful lot of my life and my thinking. And I've got a very busy life – I've got lots of friends, I do a lot of stuff – but they are the core of my life. I think about them every day.

grandmother of eight

Perhaps especially so when a loved husband has died:

My grandchildren have given me a reason to live after my husband passed away. When I got the grandchildren, I was so happy, I felt I had a reason to live now. I get up every morning thinking of them – I'm going to cook for them, or I'm going to bring them from their school, or it's half-term and they are going to come and stay with me. All the time, that keeps me going.

There are moments when I think what have I got in my life now? And there is nothing – but the next minute I think Oh, I've got the grandchildren – I feel that I'm living for them.

grandmother of four

Yet there can be a sadness from watching life take its inevitable course:

It's a little sad watching them grow older, but it's how things are. Khalil Gibran, I think, said children are the arrows – you've got the bow and the parent shoots the arrow, but they're no longer yours. They have to live their own lives. Grandparenting is a bit like that. You have to help them as the springboard to start them off and hope and pray that they will live well. That they will live and love and laugh – and care about themselves and about other people.

grandmother of two

And it can be seen as almost a secret club:

I had a lovely card from a close friend who is also a granny which said, 'Welcome to the best club in the world!' And it's just how it felt. Quite a few of us, friends who are also grannies, are just are a bit smug about it from time to time, saying 'Oh, isn't it nice to be a granny, isn't it lovely.'

There's all that business about having the best deal because you have the pleasure of the children without that relentlessness and that anxiety and responsibility. It's such a privilege and you feel such an important part of a team, you are a necessary support. When you're retired, it gives your life shape and meaning.

grandmother of two

Finally, and fundamentally, it makes a woman think about the trajectory of life:

Both becoming a grandmother and retiring – the two things at different times – each time you question the fragility of your life. You feel you are moving up, passing on. It makes you question things about life and how long you have to live.

There's another generation that has come up – and you belong to the one who would have to leave to make room. And you think, am I going to see them as adults? I'm not eternal. I'd just like to see what's going to happen.

grandmother of two

Chapter 2
Becoming a Grandmother

The first step in being a grandmother is becoming one through the birth of a baby to a son or daughter. It is totally accepted that this is a period of great excitement, combined with trepidation, for the prospective parents, but perhaps it is less well appreciated that similar emotions beset the prospective grandparents as well. This section discusses the processes of pregnancy and birth from a grandmother's point of view.

Being told about the pregnancy

Hearing the news
Grandmothers seem to remember exactly the moment when they learned that their daughter or daughter-in-law was expecting their first grandchild:

> They were going to a wedding and she was trying on a dress and my son said 'The only problem is that she looks pregnant in that one, doesn't she?' And I said no, because I thought it was an offensive thing to say. And then I added, 'She's not, is she?' and he nodded his head and she nodded, too.

> I just whooped, I jumped for joy. It had been a long time coming, because I was 63, no signs of any grandchildren, so I was absolutely delighted.
> *grandmother of one*

> They'd been married for some years, I knew that they both wanted children, it was completely in the normal order of things – but I hadn't anticipated it. So it was a shock, it took me by

surprise. My knees went out from underneath me and I slid down the wall and sat on the floor. I didn't expect to feel that kind of physical response, it was quite dramatic. You suddenly well up with some really strong feelings – excitement and joy, but also anxiety and fear for your daughter. Because having a child is such hard work. Not the labour and childbirth, but it's such a big thing to take on.

grandmother of two

News of the subsequent grandchildren is still a special moment, but it somehow has less weight:

For the second child, they gave me a present last Christmas. It's a silver and glass heart. And my son had written on it, 'Hi, Nanny, can't wait to meet you. Be here around July or August, with love from Number Two'. It was really lovely.

grandmother of one

The pregnancy may have been expected for some time:

When children get married, you do think that sooner or later you are going to be a grandmother, but we didn't talk about it much. When my daughter first got married, she said she wanted to have some time before starting a family. But after five years of her marriage, I knew that she wanted a baby.

She came in the house, her face was glowing, she had a funny smile and I knew what it was. I said, 'Is it yes?' and she said, 'Yes, I've just came from the hospital, and I wanted you to be the first to know'. I hugged both of them and said, 'Come, we'll tell Daddy.'

grandmother of four

Or it can come as a great surprise:

I'd been waiting for a long time and thought it wasn't going to happen. I can remember being about age 40 and thinking I could be a granny, because I had my children young. And twenty years later, my son was in a relationship, but it looked like they weren't interested in having children.

I wasn't pestering them every two minutes, but I was thinking about it – it was the elephant in the room. Maybe once a year, I'd say something like, 'Are you thinking, at some point, you might have children?' Something fairly tentative. My son actually said at one point I was very good at not asking all the time.

grandmother of two

My daughter has polycystic ovaries and they told her that she'd never be able to have children. And about two months after that, she said she didn't feel well, she kept being sick, and she was putting on weight. I finally asked if she was pregnant and she started crying, and said yes. She was frightened to tell me because she wasn't married. But we were pleased, we couldn't wait.

grandmother of one

Occasionally, grandparents will get involved in helping the process along:

My son and his wife thought that they couldn't have any children. They were trying for about 18 months, and began to go to various fertility people. My husband said, 'I don't care how much money it costs, I'm going to make sure that they can have a child.' He told my son to make whatever appointments they needed and he would pay for it. And while they were making all these appointments, she got pregnant.

grandmother of five

In some cases, the announcement is full of uneasiness for one reason or another:

She rang me up when she was already 20 weeks pregnant. I was a bit disappointed that she hadn't told me straight away. She wasn't married, she'd had a miscarriage the year before, and she was anticipating that I wouldn't be pleased. She was right.

It was a rather bizarre conversation – 'I'm just ringing to tell you that I'm pregnant.' 'Oh! How many weeks?' 'Twenty.' 'Oh, right, ok.' And 'Have a nice holiday – goodbye.' That was it. I was a bit shell-shocked.

grandmother of three

My daughter was 18, not married, but she had a partner. I was concerned that she was happy about it and that they would be able to cope. It was all about support, really – supporting her. There was nothing particular wrong, but you think, was it an accident? She was very happy, absolutely.

grandmother of one

For one woman, grandchildren seem to come in threes, like the proverbial buses:

> My daughter was quite young, 23, and it was out of the blue. I think he was a mistake, but a nice mistake and I was pleased for her. The following week, my other daughter rang – they'd been trying for ages, it seemed like it was never going to happen. I thought oh, we're going to have two together. And when she had her 12 week scan, we realised that she was having twins – so, three. When they were born, I went from two grandchildren to five!
>
> *grandmother of six*

Becoming a great-grandmother is even more of a shock:

> My daughter phoned and told me 'Mum, you're going to be a great-grandmum.' I said, 'What – am I?' I was happy for her. But it felt like it's not happening to *me*, I don't feel that old.
>
> *grandmother of ten*

First thoughts

Many things go through a woman's mind when she learns of a pregnancy in the next generation. There are, of course, many people to be told:

> I called my mum. She was over the moon, it was going to be her first great-grandchild. My other kids were, too. One knew before me, so when I went to tell her, she was laughing and said, 'I knew, Mum. I knew before you.' She was all excited. And then we told my seven-year-old

and he just couldn't wait. He just thought that maybe they take a pill and a baby comes.

grandmother of one

A number of grandmothers relive their own early years:

When my daughter told me that she was expecting, I felt like it's not her – *I'm* expecting! It's a very funny feeling, I went back so many years to when I was expecting her and it was like I'm going to have a baby again. I was very happy and excited, I'm going to be mum again.

grandmother of four

In some cultures, preparing for a grandchild begins very early:

Once our daughter started work, we started looking for a prospective husband for her, because that's how we do in our Indian community. We used to tell her, you've got to start thinking of getting married and having children.

My husband was worried that she should find an Indian partner. He used to pester her about always being too busy with her work. In our community, once the children are grown up, you start by word of mouth, people ask, 'Oh, your daughter's grown-up, is she interested to get married? I know a nice young person...'

grandmother of two

And the announcement has a more profound effect for some grandmothers-to-be:

I was 51. It was a shock. I think the immediate thought was I'm not ready to be a grandparent, it sounds old. I still felt that I was very busy parenting. But maybe it was just the thought of going into another phase of life, I'm moving into another generation. And it's a signifier of mortality, I suppose. That initial feeling was quite short-lived – and then I was delighted.

grandmother of three

She told me on the phone. Of course I knew she was going to have a baby, but with a lot of things that happen in your life, like the death of one's parents, you move up a rung of some ladder and you become the next stage yourself. I think maybe in the back of my mind, that's what happened – I'd moved on somehow.

grandmother of eight

Involvement in the pregnancy

Levels of involvement
Grandmothers vary in the extent to which they are involved in their daughter or daughter-in-law's pregnancies. Some live too far away or simply do not feel they are particularly needed at this point:

Her husband was a tremendous support and he's an exceptionally constant and attentive father – they didn't need me. I just watched her get terribly big. I did spend time with her, but not hugely.

grandmother of two

I was not so much involved because they lived some distance away – and I was still working.

But I went to the 20-week scan with them. Seeing the baby on the scanner was very moving – just to think there's this little extension of you inside the mum's tummy – you just can't believe it's happening.

grandmother of one

Some pay a bit more attention to the pregnant daughter or daughter-in-law than previously:

Old fashioned grandmas would cook and say you've got to eat for two now. I don't believe in all that, you don't want them to be putting on unnecessary weight. But I did take care of them. I would urge her to come and eat here. That way, I know that I've cooked a proper meal for her. I even offered to make some particular food if she fancied it.

grandmother of two

It is also a time for some discussions:

When my daughter was expecting her first child, I asked what she needed from me, because my mother had died before she was born. I therefore hadn't any experience of a mother-grandmother relationship. – I told her that we would have to learn along the way.

grandmother of two

And some are heavily involved:

I went to all her hospital appointments and all her ante-natal classes, because her husband works nights. We couldn't wait for the scan to find out whether it was a girl or a boy. She had pictures done for us of the baby and we pinned them on the board. Every time she went for a different scan, we put them on the board to see its progress.

grandmother of one

I was going out to buy the clothing, looking at prams – I was really excited. I told everyone. She had a lot of back problems and ended up coming to stay with me. I just wanted to take care of her, to make sure nothing happened. If I felt she was overdoing it a bit, I'd be urging her to sit down. It was more work for me, but I was at home anyway.

grandmother of one

Some grandmothers, even those who live a long way away, do a fair amount of worrying:

I try not to worry, but you do. It's worry more about my child than the baby. The mother is your child and until the baby comes, it's the mother you're very concerned about. They're still your children.

With one, they thought the baby was Down's Syndrome and my daughter was in a terrible state. We discussed would she have a termination, but she decided she wouldn't. She paid for a special test – and it turned out she wasn't Down's Syndrome after all. In fact, she's a very bright little girl.

grandmother of eleven

And some save little mementoes from this period:

She went for a few scans and I went with her – it was really exciting. At her first one, the 12 weeks, we got all the little scan photos. We put the scans up on little photo frames and in my purse. We got a few for the family and handed them out as well.

grandmother of one

My son had been told he has a low sperm count and he would probably never have children, but then she got pregnant. Just took a pregnancy test out of the pound shop, the little thing with the pink stripe down it. I've still got it upstairs, put away.

grandmother of two

Giving advice
The traditional mother probably gave a lot of advice to her pregnant daughter or daughter-in-law. Current mothers appear to be more cautious about this, often because they see their children getting advice elsewhere:

I'm pretty sure she got a lot of information on what to expect from professionals – 'always expect the unexpected' sort of thing. Nurses, all the maternity team, those kind of people. I was never a knitting baby clothes kind of person – I can't knit. I just wanted to do whatever she wanted me to do and to help in any way I could.

grandmother of one

She's a very tough, independent young woman. We're not the sort of mother and daughter who ring each other every morning. I suppose she did talk about things, but I was more of a long-stop.

She talked more to friends of her own age, who had had children, and people she met along the way at these NCT classes. I wasn't her main source of advice.

grandmother of two

And it is partly because much advice changes hugely from one era to another:

If they asked me something, I would say what I think, but it's so different with kids today. They mustn't ever drink, they mustn't eat certain cheeses. And I thought, well, I had all that and there's nothing wrong with my kids. So, what is it with them today? My mum was forever telling me not to do this, not to do that – what I was doing was wrong. I've never did that with mine.

grandmother of eight

A recurrent theme in grandmothers' stories is the difference in their relationships with the families of their daughters and those of their sons. This starts at the point of pregnancy. Mothers of sons often seem to be less involved than mothers of daughters:

I've never had a very easy relationship with my son – well, on and off. But there was nothing I could do, apart from saying that it was all going to be fine. As the pregnancy developed, I became concerned for her health, but I don't think I gave much advice. Her mum was more involved. That was okay with me, I recognised that she wanted to be closer to her mother at that time.

grandmother of three

But, where needed, a mother-in-law will step into the breach:

> I was involved with my daughter-in-law, because her mum wasn't. She wasn't very close to her mum at the time, so she really relied on me. I felt honoured. Like I was the one who went with her to the hospital appointments, I was with her at the birth.
>
> *grandmother of six*

The birth

Helping out

Grandmothers who do not live near their children necessarily have to wait for the news of the birth of a grandchild. But those who live nearby can find themselves very involved. Some play an unexpectedly important role:

> Near her due date, she couldn't feel the baby move. I took her to the hospital – his heartbeat kept dropping and they were quite concerned and booked her in for the next day. By eleven the following night, it still hadn't happened. I knew from the readings that it was not right, and asked the nurse why was the baby's heart dropping? She went right away to get the doctor, who said she needed an emergency Caesarean. If I hadn't taken her to the hospital the night before, I would not have known whether that was low or high. I wouldn't have taken any notice.
>
> It was really scary in the Caesarean room, there were just so many people. All of a sudden, you see this baby come up in the air – but there was

no sound. The nurses were putting little tubes in him and pumping him and I was panicking – he's not crying, he's just laying there. My daughter's putting her hands out to me and saying, 'What's happening?' Then suddenly, they picked him up, did a few turns and he gave out a big scream. We found out later that she'd had Pethidine and it will put a baby to sleep.

grandmother of one

We got to the hospital and they said we had to wait in a waiting room, she was getting quite bad by then, but she'd only been in labour for about two hours – because it was her first, they thought she was going to be a long time. She started being sick, in front of all the people, and I lost my rag, and said, 'I think she should be somewhere a bit private.'

They examined her and she was ready to go. After that, it was just go, go, go – so quick, she was only four hours. I was able to stay in the delivery room until the morning. We all stayed, that was lovely. None of us had any sleep.

grandmother of six

And one tells how she found herself delivering the baby:

My son's partner asked me if I would be there, because her mother couldn't. They had discussed it and decided they would like for me to be there. I felt very honoured – I'd never been at a birth other than my own giving birth, so I was thrilled. Waiting was difficult, just being there for all those hours and not really knowing how involved to be – when to stand back, when to come forward. I wondered if she felt it was a mistake to have me there, because I was kind of standing there, not knowing how do I contribute to this, but not intrude.

Right at the end, I was on the floor with the midwife and my son's partner was kind of squatting and he was behind her, holding her and the midwife said, 'Come on, Granny. You're going to deliver your grandchild.' And the partner was saying, 'Come on.' and it was so lovely.

It was an amazing honour. The midwife was with me, holding my wrists firmly, because they were slightly shaking – it was absolutely incredible. My granddaughter came out, I took her in my hands and I gave her to my son's partner and my son. Absolutely wonderful.

grandmother of three

The difference between daughters and sons emerges again here:

It was me, her mum and my son at the hospital. It was my grandchild going to be born, but it was a different being my son's partner, because she was crying for her mum, whereas when it was my daughters, they were crying for me. When you're in pain you want your mum.

Once the baby was born, they let me wash and dress the baby and I put her in her first babygro. It feels important to be the first one that's dressed them. Her mum was with her, she was needing her mum. So, I got the baby.

grandmother of six

Some women find that they are not as helpful as they might have expected:

During the early stages of labour, I was very good at supporting her and doing the right things. But as soon as the midwife came in – and therefore somebody else became responsible – I completely went to pieces. If I could've paced up and down the corridor and smoked sixteen packets of fags, I would have done. I more or less sat in a chair and whimpered 'Oh, no, oh, no.' Which is strange because, beforehand, I thought that I would always be there for her when she needed me. It was just total meltdown. There were things about me that I didn't know. Happily, her sister turned up and took over as helpmate through labour.

It's a terrible thing to witness your child, your most treasured person, in such pain. And there is an element of serious risk. So seeing her going through the painful contractions was quite harrowing and there was massive anxiety in case something went wrong. You don't know what condition the baby's going to be in, you don't know what condition the mother's going to be in. And when it's your own – just don't be there, it's awful, really awful.

The second time, we all agreed that I stay at home. I looked after the first one, my other daughter went with them and his mum was close

by. I saw her the next morning. It was lovely –
my lovely daughter sitting up in bed, perfectly all
right with this brand-new, gorgeous baby. It was
a huge relief. I was really grateful that I'd been
spared the anxiety of being there.

grandmother of two

And some feel a bit excluded from the process:

At the last minute, my daughter's husband
persuaded her to have a Caesarean. I found that
absolutely shocking – I had been preparing her
for a natural birth and I felt cheated. While we
were all waiting, he was very intrusive – in every
step, he was there to tell me to shut up.

I wasn't present at the delivery. He was
absolutely territorial about the whole thing,
protecting the room and my daughter and saying
it was only him that would be present during the
birth. I thought how much have I been robbed of
my pleasure seeing my daughter give birth? I
felt absolutely dismissed.

grandmother of two

Seeing the baby for the first time
For grandparents, as well as parents, this is a time of
heightened emotion:

It was lovely. I didn't actually cry, but I did feel
really overwhelmed and it was much more of a
feeling than I had anticipated. When you've just
had your own child, you're a little bit involved in
delivering the baby, whereas it was just like a
present. And he looked lovely because he didn't

have any marks on his face, so he looked very handsome.

grandmother of five

It is blissful and hugely surprising. When I first held my own daughter, it was a real shock. I thought I would get a blank piece of paper that you would write on. But when she came out, she took one look at me and I thought, oh my God, it's a complete stranger, this is somebody I don't know. And when I first held my little granddaughter, I thought, here we go again – here's another one. There's a whole new person. And that was a huge delight.

grandmother of two

One woman describes simply hearing the news:

My son rang me in the middle of the night, when they were on their way to the hospital, and I asked if they wanted me to come, but he said no. I think they wanted to be just together and that was fine. The next morning, he phoned, 'It's a little girl, mum, she's really beautiful', I couldn't believe it.

I was a librarian and you should be quiet in the library, but I just said loudly, 'No, really!' I was just jumping up and down and I had to go outside. We were so pleased.

grandmother of one

And this is a moment when the fact of being a grandmother finally hits home:

A message came through to me at work telling me that the baby was born, and I went straight to the hospital. I had to ring a bell and somebody asked me who I was and I remember saying, 'I'm the *grandmother* – so let me in.' I felt they couldn't possibly leave me at the door! I had some rights.

grandmother of two

The first weeks

Grandmothers have a number of roles in the first weeks after the birth of a baby.

Helping the new mother
A few grandmothers find themselves heavily involved when their daughter – or occasionally daughter-in-law – comes home from hospital:

I used to go every day, because she was living not far away. I'd go to see how she was doing and help her. If she was having a bath, I used to sit with him. It was lovely. My mind was going back to when I was looking after my own child – how it was in the hospital, how I was scared sometimes to handle her. It's like my daughter has become small now and I'm bringing her up.

grandmother of four

From the day she became pregnant, I knew that I was going to look after him. And once he was born, I was the mother, I took care of the baby. I did everything. I did the cleaning, the washing, everything. In Nigeria, when your daughter has a child, it is expected that you do all that.

grandmother of three

The occasional grandmother may make herself very useful, even when the mother is still in hospital:

The baby caught a bit of jaundice and they put her under this special incubator light – every twenty minutes you had to keep feeding her and turning her. Because my daughter had had a Caesarean, she couldn't lift the baby, so I stayed all night – taking her out, feeding her, and just making sure that she was fine. I think it has affected my bond with her.

grandmother of one

My daughter was 17. It was different times then – they took the babies away from you and put them into a nursery. Because she had to have a blood transfusion, she wasn't able to go down and see the baby, so I used to go down to visit. When she was finally able to get up to see the baby, the nurse said, 'No, the mother's already been.' They thought I was the mother, because I was going down each day to see him. It was like he was another one of mine. That bond was there right from the beginning.

grandmother of seven

Sometimes, a daughter may come back to live with her mother or parents. Many grandmothers really enjoy reliving the days of having a baby in the house:

She came back to me and stayed about a month. It was really nice because I was able to deal with him, so she could get some sleep. She'd got an infection, so people would come out to her a few times in the week, to re-dress it all. It was better for me to take the baby and feed him and bath him. I felt like a mum all over again. I had to keep telling myself – you're the nan, you're not the mum.

grandmother of one

After one night in hospital, she wanted to come home. So I made up her room here, and put the baby cot and everything in it. In India, where I come from, it's the custom for the daughter to go home to her mother for the first forty days after delivery. That first night, she was very tired and I told her to get some sleep, I would look after him.

I went to the spare bedroom, I took this baby and put him on my chest, and I spent the whole night holding him. I couldn't put him down because the cot was in her room. I didn't sleep. It was just so great.

She stayed with me for six weeks and I virtually brought up the baby during that time – she hardly did anything. I told her that once she went home, she would have to take over, so take it easy now, enjoy it while she could. And she said 'Oh, you can carry on, Mum.'

grandmother of two

Early signs of problems

Problems can begin in families from a very early stage, even soon after birth:

She was having a home birth. My son wasn't the type to ring and say that she had just gone into labour or it's four hours in – I didn't have any communication at all. I just happened to ring – and she'd just given birth! I said, 'All right then.' So I was kept in the dark. I would never have pushed for more access, because I don't like confrontation. If someone clearly doesn't want to give you something, it wouldn't help to push yourself.

grandmother of three

I wasn't very emotional about the first baby because she was so tiny – she was four weeks premature and my daughter was all hyper. She was such a difficult person at that time. I went to see her after she gave birth and she thought I wasn't there at the right time and didn't give her enough attention.

And there was a big argument about the name. They had a list of names and I said I really liked one of them and she insisted 'None of your business – *we're* going to decide!' So, I thought, I better not interfere with this lot.

grandmother of two

Problems may also manifest themselves in the early weeks:

After my daughter had gone home from hospital, I cooked her a very nice herb soup which makes the milk more abundant when a woman is breastfeeding. It is a Middle Eastern thing. But the whole of the casserole was left out on the doorstep. Her husband didn't want it in his house, he has got a special sensitivity towards anything cultural.

grandmother of two

When my daughter-in-law and I went out when her first daughter was born, I was the proud grandmother, pushing the pram. Several people stopped and asked if it was my baby and I had to say, no, it's my granddaughter. By the end of the day, she had the hump – she said it comes to something when the grandmother gets more remarks than the mother! I felt like it was a competition between me and her. It's not so much an issue now, I've aged a bit.

grandmother of two

The parents were very protective and we didn't see the baby for at least a fortnight – they were following their own idea about how to bond with the baby. So it was difficult, the first few weeks. But they were delighted, it was a gorgeous baby – a big very healthy boy, absolutely fine.

Once my son had gone back to work, I would go there about once a week. But it would be to be with her to help, to hold the baby, change the nappy every now and again, but not to take charge of the baby myself at all. I don't know why. We used to joke, perhaps she thinks that we don't know how to do it.

grandmother of two

Chapter 3
Doing Things Together

A major part of being a grandmother is having some contact with the grandchildren, doing things together and simply having fun. In this chapter, grandmothers talk about their activities with their grandchildren, from the day-to-day to large family get-togethers and holidays.

Levels of involvement
The extent to which grandmothers are involved with their grandchildren depends in part on how close they live to each other and the needs of the family.

Regular arrangements
In young families, it is quite common for there to be a regular arrangement, often a day a week, for grandmothers to take over. Sometimes this is to enable the daughter or daughter-in-law to work, helping to save the high costs of childcare:

> You find grandmothers tend to have their grandchildren more than they ever did, because the nursery fees are exorbitant. I've had more involvement since my daughter went back to work. I have the granddaughter once a week. It saves them money having even the one day.
>
> *grandmother of one*

> She went back to work after six months and I looked after the baby, while she was at work. It was just lovely having a baby again in the house. I just love babies – they're so clingy to you, they need you, they're just so helpless.
>
> *grandmother of six*

But it can also be because of uneasiness about any other form of childcare:

I'm like a full-time mum, because my daughter's gone back to work and we look after the baby during the day. We feed and change her and if my daughter's working late, we get her all bathed and ready. So when she gets home from work, she can spend some time before she puts her to bed.

She told us that if she didn't have us as grandparents, she wouldn't have gone back to work, because she wouldn't have trusted anybody else. She felt safe that we'd look after the baby and that we'd do it really well.

grandmother of one

When I went to work, I had to use a baby minder and it was terrible, there were no council regulations in those days. My daughter can still tell me things. So, when she wanted to go back to work, I said was that there no way she would send her child to any nursery or baby minder – I would look after him. She used to bring him at seven in the morning. We had a cot, we had everything.

And sometimes they would come late to get him because my son-in-law works pretty late. They would eat here and then I would tell them there was no point in taking him home at ten at night to bring him back the next day at seven.

grandmother of two

Where a grandmother has more than one set of grandchildren, arrangements can become very complicated:

The younger ones, we look after every Tuesday. I collect the little one from nursery and we collect another from school. I give both of them dinner, and by then my daughter's usually home. And another two, I'm now collecting on a Thursday. I've always looked after the grandchildren a day a week. At one point, I couldn't physically manage them all – they don't live in the same area and I couldn't fit four in the car. I had a double buggy.

grandmother of eleven

But sometimes, these arrangements are more for the grandparents:

When she was about 12 months old, my partner and I used to take her every Sunday for lunch. She loved spaghetti, so we used to go to spaghetti houses and I still remember her sitting in a high chair and her face covered with sauce. At one point we were told by her parents that *they* would like to see her on Sunday, too, so we had to slow down a bit. We would've liked to carry on, but we could understand that they wanted to see her.

grandmother of two

Some younger grandmothers have young children at the same time as their children, so they all play together:

I could go to my daughter's house and she would have everything I needed because the boys were of a similar age. It was just brilliant. The children of my friends were all grown up, so this gave us a nice bond. My son goes off and plays with her kids and my daughter and I just sit and chat. I've even stayed there overnight, when needed.

grandmother of three

But one grandmother describes how she isn't needed so much, because of the involvement of the father:

I'm not involved so much, because they have got a very good bond, my daughter and her partner, and he's very hands-on with the nappies and all. To me, it's unusual because in my time men didn't, it was all down to the mum.

grandmother of six

Living together
In contrast, some grandchildren live with their grandparents or grandmother if she is on her own, either full-time or off and on. This makes for different sorts of relationships:

Children and grandchildren, it's the same, I brought two of the grandchildren up – I washed, I cooked, I did everything for them. I would take the boy to and from school. If he's not well, he won't go to his mum – he comes to me. Even his mum will say, 'They're *your* children.'

When my daughter had her boy, she was having a tough time with an alcoholic man – I said she might as well come live with me, not knowing that he would come as well. Her man would come in drunk and I looked after the grandkids, because I didn't want them to suffer. Eventually, I couldn't take it any more, so he moved out and she is still here with the two kids.

grandmother of ten

I had them living with me till she was about three, because they couldn't get a council flat. It was lovely. Although they were living with me, his partner's mother used to have them every weekend. So, for two days, the grandchild was at her other nan's.

grandmother of eight

One grandmother recounts how she brought up her grandson on her own:

When my daughter went to America with her new husband, I kept the boy here in London. We would go on holidays to see her, but he went to primary and secondary school here. I was both mum and dad to this boy and I often thought of him as my son. I had done it once and the second time was not hard. I taught him how to do his own bed, to cook, wash up, hoover the place. He learned to go and buy things, he learned to take the initiative in things.

grandmother of three

Living together may also be solely for particular periods because of the needs of the family:

In the early years, I was *very* involved. My granddaughter used to stay overnight from when she was six months or so. There was tremendous trust that I could look after their child. My son was a successful musician and he was often off touring around the world. The women and children of his group were left at home. It was very sad, I could see he became very drained, but I helped them a lot.

grandmother of two

Living together is not always easy:

They need to be in London but can't afford a house of their own, so they asked to stay here, very reluctantly. She didn't really want to come to live with us. I wasn't keen on sharing my home with her either. I wanted to do my own thing and all of a sudden she said, 'I'm coming to stay.' My heart cried, but I didn't tell her.

She wanted things her way. For example, in the evening she doesn't want anyone coming to the house – or even the phone to ring – because her daughter is going to be disturbed. But it's my home! I had to do a lot of adjusting, but she thinks that she's done the adjusting. I had to give up my social life.

grandmother of two

Distant grandchildren

But there are many grandmothers who see their grandchildren much less often. This happens, of course, where they do not live nearby. Of course, many grandmothers try to visit as often as convenient to the family:

One family lives just out of London. I go out at least once a month and usually spend Christmas with them. The relationship with that family is pretty good – they've got a family that seems to run like a family should, you can sit and have a coffee and chat to the children and just feel a part of life. I think I'm part of their lives, which I like. I'm sure it does make a difference in how you relate.

grandmother of eight

My daughter was living in America when she had twin babies and her husband had left her. She phoned and begged me to come to help. I would go there for three months, because I can go for 90 days with a British passport, I would come back – and then maybe a week later I would go back. There's no year I don't go to America, at least once or twice. I am very close to them. I enjoy doing it, but sometimes, I do find it a bit tiring.

grandmother of three

Some family relationships are very strained, in addition to the distance:

My younger son had separated early on from the mother of his children, who lived abroad. He had been abusive – and threatening – to me for years and I became very frightened. It was heart-breaking, but eventually we went to court and there was a restraining order. I wanted him to know that I wasn't going to put up with that any more. His twin girls were just age three.

I made a decision that I would maintain a relationship with his partner, because I thought the children should know who their grandmother is, especially as he doesn't see them now and they don't see the rest of the family. And I wanted to know them.

I went recently to visit them and it was a bit stressful, but also nice. I cooked and tidied and I made some clothes for one of their dolls. They're interested in me, but they keep me at a distance, partly because they don't speak English. I think also because I'm their dad's mum and there were difficulties with him. This time was a bit better. One will lean on me and the other will sidle up to me and sort of sniff me out, and by the end of the stay, it's relaxed a bit. I try to fit in and hang on in there, but I get upset and I come back in tears.

grandmother of three

One family lives further away. They're lovely grandchildren, but I was not as involved as much as I would have liked, partly because of the distance, but also because the parents were not getting on well and it was a bit awkward staying with them. There was an uncomfortable atmosphere and I didn't go there more often because of that.

I wasn't quite sure how to manage it. You can't go and be critical, but seeing things not going right – that's life and that's bound to happen – but it's very hard to watch in people you love. And because I saw them much more seldom, I felt more of a visitor there than as part of the set-up.

grandmother of eight

Some find they have to make an effort to keep in touch:

> I moved not long ago. When I still lived in our family home, I used to see the grandchildren regularly. In the first couple of months after I moved, I didn't see them very much, but I missed them. So I'm now making more of an effort – 'Oh, I haven't seen you since last Friday, just wondered if I could pop over one evening? Shall we do supper and I'll come and bathe the kids?' And so we're beginning to get a different working pattern.
>
> ***grandmother of two***

And some virtually lose contact for one reason or another:

> Since one of my children went to live in Spain, it's years since I've seen them. It's hard. One son is not together with the children's mum anymore – they'd still let me see the grandkids, but I don't, she won't talk to me. I will send gifts, but I don't see them. I would love to, though, because they're getting big now – one of them is 12.
>
> ***grandmother of ten***

> When they were younger, I was around my children and grandchildren a lot, but as they've got older, the partners changed, and they moved away. My youngest son has three children, but he's married to somebody else now, so I see those children hardly ever. Some grandchildren I might only see them four times in ten years. I've

got about three or four great-grandchildren on the way this year.

grandmother of seven

Activities with grandchildren
What grandmothers do when they are with their grandchildren varies enormously, of course, with the age of the child.

Babies and toddlers
Babies and toddlers are fairly straight forward. Grandmothers find many things to do in the home as well as outside:

> I just remember sitting on the floor and playing with puzzles and things. She loves to learn – as a baby, she was just drinking up everything that you would put in front of her – music, anything. Her mother has always done a lot of drawing with her and even when she was very little, she would look at things and say, 'Look at the texture or the colour of this.' She amazed me.
>
> *grandmother of two*

> I play with him, talk with him, he loves books. He's got a garage, we play cars, he likes you to watch films and DVDs. And, of course, now he's started talking, he copies everything you say, so you've got to be careful what you say. Daren't ever swear with him around, because he will say it.
>
> *grandmother of eight*

> I have a friend who is the grandmother of a two-year old as well and we meet. In the winter, there's quite a nice little area in the library where

the little ones can have a little read and a play with the toys. In the summer, it's easier because you can take them out and they'll run around for ages and play. We take them down to the duck pond and feed the ducks.

grandmother of one

Some grandmothers do have problems, however:

He is a heavy baby. My back is aching all the time. I should know when to say I cannot do something, especially lifting. I should create facilities in my environment so that I don't have to lift him. I would be happier if I could move without pain.

grandmother of one

Young grandchildren

As babies grow into children, many grandmothers come into their own. They describe how they can pass hours with small children:

They've always had loads of books. We gave a love of reading to both of our kids and they have passed that on – and being inquisitive about things. We've always believed that education is really important, so we've always read to them and read poetry. I know loads of children's songs and it's fun to sing with them.

grandmother of five

I always did painting and drawing with the grandkids, cutting out and making things. And I'd have cardboard, ribbons and things, and get them to make a birthday card for their parent's birthday or something coming up. Or, we'd get them all singing and dancing. They'd climb up on the chair and do their turn – singing or telling a joke – and they'd get their applause.

grandmother of seven

I do enjoy letting my three-year-old grandson stand at the sink with me. He'll put on the tap and play with the water and the bubbles. And he cooks with me. I make him stand on the chair and I'll say, 'Look, you use this spice and that spice and this and that,' and he watches and then I let him do it himself. I give him a teaspoon, so he'll have motor skills.

I just believe that the first five years are so important – it's good to develop the child's senses – the touching, feeling, all those are important.

grandmother of one

We have treasure hunts, when we go for a walk or we're going to school. It was really weird one day, because I said, 'Come on, we're looking for treasure' and then I found a medal! It was a Mason's medal – apparently somebody got robbed and they threw it away. But, my granddaughter thinks I'm magic.

grandmother of two

Some grandmothers are very clever at creating games from very little:

Something had come in a box. I said we shouldn't take it away. That box became a garage, it became a house – all kinds of different things they played in it until it broke. And then I got the scissors and the paints and we cut out things. We made robots, houses, trees. They loved it. Children love a cardboard box.

grandmother of two

She would use the furniture and create games for herself. I can't remember how old she was, but there was a sofa that was to be thrown away. She started using it and it became part of whatever game she was playing. The sofa stayed there for years. I thought about getting rid of it, but kept thinking, no, she wants to play with it. It stayed there six or seven years more than she ever wanted to play with it.

grandmother of one

We have a big cloth, it's see-through, sort of sparkly, with different colours and broad stripes and checks on it. It's probably about six feet by four. It's been a river, a zebra crossing, it's been a tent many times, it's been wrapped round as a cloak. Their imaginative play is wonderful. That probably cost two or three pounds.

grandmother of two

And some ideas don't work:

We used to have poetry evenings with my children, which they loved, but I have not been able to carry on with my grandchildren. I've tried it, but I've failed. I used to get all the children together and put food on the table and each one would read a poem and then they could help themselves to food. I think I have lost the knack. They've got to enjoy the poem, they've got to have the whole evening, they've got to be at the age when poetry means something. Maybe they're still too young.

grandmother of five

This is often a time when grandmothers can let themselves go and have fun:

My granddaughter had some funny bouncing thing that someone gave her – you stand on it, and then you bounce up and down. I was bouncing with her. My grandson started laughing and said, 'Oh, *you* can't do it!' I told him, 'Let me do things as long as I can, because one day I'll be old and you'll have to look after me. So *then* you can laugh.'

grandmother of two

Three of the grandchildren were playing up. My daughters were also here and we put music on and started singing and dancing and clapping about. The grandchildren were looking at us and couldn't believe what was going on. One said 'What are *you* doing? You're doing what *we* should be doing!' We stopped them right in their tracks!

grandmother of seven

But some grandmothers feel they miss the opportunity to play as much as they would like:

When the parents first brought them here, I'd expected they'd take the opportunity of putting their feet up and letting granny and grandpa play with the grandchildren. But they would come, we would slave in the kitchen, and they would play with the children in our house.

I would love to say, 'You sit down, read the paper, and we'll take them for a walk'. There's a local playground we could take them to. But it's always *with* the parents – they need to be in charge of whatever interaction there is.

grandmother of two

Older grandchildren

As children grow into teenagers, they lead their own lives and it becomes harder for grandmothers to see them very frequently. Nonetheless, they can still have a role. Some take an interest in what their grandchildren are doing in school or university:

I sit with them if they have to do any notes for projects. My granddaughter had a World War Two project last term and I used to do research for her. And she asked me to teach her how to embroider and I've taught her how to do knitting.

grandmother of two

One's studying history at university and we often talk about that. She wants to know if I've got the books here that she's studying or we discuss her work. She does a lot of youth work and we sometimes talk about that or about how other things are going.

grandmother of eleven

And some find other things they like to do:

Sometimes on weekends, they might come for the day. We might go walking or might go to the large shopping centre nearby. I can't seem to get my bearings when I go there, but the kids like to go there, especially the 16-year-old.

grandmother of ten

I'm always altering her clothes, making everything tighter or higher or something has got to be changed. I bought her a handbag and she wanted me to lengthen the straps – it's these kinds of projects. I'm so grateful because without that, I think she'd be rushing off. But she comes with a bag with stuff for me to fix. It's very much to do with the physical closeness and involvement.

And I do all her Christmas shopping with her. We go out, have dinner, and we get the stuff for her parents, her friends and her other grandmother. That's lovely. It's become a regular thing. I don't give her money during the year, and then at Christmas, I'll have £100 or so and I say, 'You can use that for getting gifts for your parents and special people.'

grandmother of three

Or they note that grandchildren pop by when they want something:

Having teenage grandchildren is all right. Mostly, knock on wood, I never had any trouble with them. They're well-mannered, know to behave themselves on the street and things like that. They're good kids, but I could only talk for today, I don't know about for tomorrow. Last Friday, the 16 year-old-was here, 'You know how you love me, Nan...?' I said, 'Yes, you can have it.'

grandmother of ten

But it is also clearly the case that teenage grandchildren's interest may wane:

I'll ring up and ask if they are coming to dinner and the older one will say he's not coming tonight. If I ask why, he'll say he has too much homework, but he probably thinks it's boring coming to his grandmother. He denies it. He's a very bright kid and he's very independent.

grandmother of two

Sometimes I feel that she doesn't *really* want to see me and then I think she does. I feel a bit concerned and that I might lose her. I don't know quite how to manage this new stage of her as a bigger girl. But she's very affectionate to me, it's lovely, but I'm still adjusting to that teenage thing – she's taller than me and it's a hell of a big change.

grandmother of three

Even before they reach their teens, granny is often much less welcome:

When I was visiting them, they would all go to a life-saving club – they're in different groups. I watched the little one the first Sunday I was there, I watched the middle one the next week. I said to the 11-year-old that I would go to his group the following week – and he said, '*Don't* go anywhere near the group, I don't want anyone to know that my grandmother's watching me!' Well, it's not 'cool'.

grandmother of five

Grown-up grandchildren

Only a few grandmothers in this book have grown-up grandchildren. They generally keep in touch, one way or another:

> My oldest one kept at a slight distance, but, he's suddenly much more able to talk – he comes and does the garden for me once a week in the summer. We have lunch and we chat about his trips abroad or other things. It's a separate relationship now, outside his home environment. He likes to come, his godmother told me that. It's lovely. I'm really pleased that he wants to come and see me.
>
> *grandmother of eight*

> I take the older ones out for lunch, often together. It's a nice way of sitting and talking to them. And we take them to the theatre two or three times a year, if I find something that I think is suitable.
>
> *grandmother of eleven*

> I don't want them to come to see me because it's duty – I want them to come because they *want* to. In fact, they'll phone me up and they'll say, 'Grandma, we're getting a macaroni cheese withdrawal' because they love my macaroni cheese. I can't cook, but I've got my own recipe and they all love it. It's comfort food.
>
> *grandmother of two*

> One grandchild's been in my life all of her life. She practically lives with me and she stays here unless she's at her boyfriend's. She looks on me as her mum, really. She didn't get on too well

with her mother – she says, 'I can't talk to Mummy, but I can talk to you.' She pops in for clothes to be washed or to ask me to do something. I don't mind. She sometimes will bring me a bunch of flowers.

grandmother of eight

One grandmother has a family that has a lot of fun together. She describes her daughter's recent wedding to her longstanding partner, when the grandchildren were already grown up:

My daughter didn't get married until about five years ago. I had forgotten they weren't married. It was in a registry office, with just the immediate family. It was the best wedding I've been to, because nobody could stop giggling. At one point, the registrar asked if I could please control them.

While they were signing the register, my oldest granddaughter piped up, 'Oh my God, Grandma, does this mean we're legitimate now?' Everybody roared, including the registrar.

grandmother of two

Coping with lots of grandchildren

A few grandmothers have very large numbers of grandchildren and it might seem to be a job in itself to keep track of them. But those in this situation do not find it overwhelming:

I don't think of the ten of them as 'a whole'. I think of them individually when they're coming to stay, when they're having birthdays – or if they've just got through school or something has happened.

Or you may think, I haven't spoken to the youngest in some time – next time I ring, I must remember to ask how her music lessons are going.

I'm not constantly thinking of them, but it tends to cluster around birthdays or exams or some significant thing that's happening.

grandmother of ten

With my eleven grandchildren, I have a diary by the phone. It is our family calendar and everybody's birthday is on there – everybody at least gets a card and the children all get presents. There's ages on there so that we can remember. I never forget my grandchildren or my children's birthdays.

I like having a lot of grandchildren and we feel there's always room for another one. I was one of five, so I am used to a big family.

grandmother of eleven

Having a very large family enables grandmothers to enjoy different ages at the same time:

They're lovely at all stages. At the moment, we've got the new baby, but I also love the teenage girls who are always in love with somebody, like Benedict Cumberbatch, or who love shopping expeditions. And the boys, similarly. Each stage brings its pleasures.

grandmother of ten

It's easier with the older ones, rather than babies or toddlers. It's less physical, because you don't have to watch them. It's much more about chatting with them and feeding them. The much older grandchildren move on to another life – it's a different relationship with them than it is with younger ones.

grandmother of eleven

Family get-togethers
Big family get-togethers can be fun and grandmothers in some cultures make these a regular event:

On holy days and Passover, we all come together, plus my sisters and their grandchildren and children. We're getting a bit big now, so we often split up for one of the days. Friday nights – not every week, but often – and on main festivals, we all get together. For the New Year, we always have one of the days when we all lunch together at one daughter's house, because they are observant, so they won't drive.

grandmother of eleven

They will meet here on Diwali, Christmastime, whenever there are bank holidays. We make a point that the whole family should get together during school holidays, either at my house or my daughter's house. On birthdays, we all are out together there. It makes me very, very, happy when they are here. Sometimes, the children play around in the house, they go and jump in my bed. They are enjoying my house. I feel that my house is smiling.

grandmother of four

Some are more conscious of the tiring aspects:

One Christmas, the whole family came together – it was fun, but oh my God, I just wanted them to go home. There were too many of them, with my children and the grands – the house was full. My children do the cooking and I put my feet up. They come for two days.

But when they're gone, it's a huge relief. I can have too much of running up and down the stairs and the noise – screaming, yelling 'She's eating all of this,' 'I didn't get any of that.' kind of thing.

grandmother of ten

Sometimes it's a bit of a struggle, because you're trying to cook a meal for everybody, you're wanting to play with the children, you're wanting to have a relaxed time – and something has to give. We recently had a lovely afternoon when we went to their house and brought the lunch with us. We went with a big chicken casserole, handed it over, so we had a lot more time to chat with everybody.

grandmother of two

For older grandmothers, family get-togethers have a special meaning of bringing their progeny all in the same place:

Family gatherings do happen from time to time. For me, it's lovely to have them all together. My great grandchild came to my 80th birthday, so they were all there. I very much wanted the different sets of grandchildren to get together, because the family means a lot. They're much of an age, a lot of them, and my hope always is that everybody will get on and be there for each other.

grandmother of eight

In my old age, I'm doing my best to remind my children to keep in touch, phone your cousin, get all the family together. My children don't care – I'm the one who is pushing it. In my past, I had a wonderful Christmas, with a long, long, table – twenty-six of us – with we, the children, being at one end, and then being very tired and sleepy.

I repeated these family gatherings in our house. Now, it's not repeating again, the numbers are halved we have to share with other in-laws.

grandmother of five

The subject of family get-togethers can be a difficult one for some grandmothers. In some cases, this is simply due to distance:

We haven't all been together as a family since a big family holiday three years ago. It was good for my husband's mother, who could see all of her great-grandchildren together. I thought the kids mightn't spend much time with her, but she was perfectly happy to just sit quietly and watch them swim or play, on the periphery. I thought, maybe that's what happens as you get older, you sort of draw back. We were in the pool with the kids – and she was just happy to sit in the shade.

grandmother of five

But it can also be due to the complexities of family dynamics:

I'd love a family get-together, but it never happens, because my son-in-law won't come here. He doesn't like mixing with anybody apart from his own family. My daughter and my grandsons come here for Christmas lunch. It's a foregone conclusion that every half term I go and see them, but there's nothing like that with my other daughter.

grandmother of three

I mostly see the grandchildren on their own, without the parents. I prefer that, because it's always very tense when they all come up together. It's the whole dynamic of the family. My son can become overprotective of the kids, doesn't want them out of his sight and can be quite dictatorial – his property, his children.

I find it really hard to be with them when it's like that. When they are with me on their own, they're fine.

grandmother of three

Holidays together
A few families also go on holiday together. In the occasional family, this is a large event:

We all take a holiday together – twenty of us, now twenty-one. Sometimes we go to a hotel. We have no rules, they don't have to stay with us all day, but it is a condition that we all eat together. We rented villas in Italy with these enormous tables like you see in the Godfather films. You sit outside to eat out in the day or night. It's lovely they all want to come. Some years, we haven't gone away because another grandchild was due, but the next year, the grandchildren said, 'When are we all going away?' It makes a warm relationship for everyone when you're away together.

grandmother of eleven

I often take a house in France and that's been great. It's very difficult to find a place, because it has to be downstairs and it has to have a proper shower room that the disabled grandson can use. Houses that are big enough to house the family – and some friends who like to come too – are few and far between.

We found one where there's a river running past the front door and you can go on a little boat or jump off a rope and swim. I never jumped off a rope, but I went on the boat. It's warm and relaxed and everybody's having a good time.

grandmother of eight

Some grandmothers take just one or two grandchildren away:

The older grandson and I are mates. I chuck him in the camper van and take him away on little trips, just me and him. We've done it a couple of times, now, starting when he was five.

We had a little chat beforehand. I said, 'You know I don't like small whiny children – but I do enjoy being with you when you're being a really nice person. You'll have to be grown-up – eat what's there and do what we need to do, because there aren't any choices – it's very small, you've got your corner, I've got mine.' It's great – we have a whale of a time.

grandmother of two

But not all such holidays are a success:

One Christmas, when my granddaughter was 15, I took the whole family on a cruise. She didn't want to come and she never spoke to any of us for three weeks. At the end, she said we'd ruined her life. I was really furious with her, because she was spoiling it for everybody.

It turned out she had some boy that she liked and there was some other girl that she thought would move in when she was away. It was nothing after three months. But she didn't open up and tell anybody. She probably had all these hormones swimming around.

grandmother of two

Keeping in touch
For some grandmothers, whose grandchildren live at a distance, there is no choice but to write or to talk on Skype or on the phone:

I email them, discussing something like a film I've seen. It's just a keeping in touch device. I do phone them from time to time, but it's not the way they communicate with each other. And it means that they have to pull themselves out of what they're doing.

If I'm in touch with them, they get back in touch with me very quickly. If I'm not, they won't unless it's my birthday or something. It's fine –

they're living their lives and I'm living mine and I know we're fond of each other and if we needed more contact, we'd have it.

grandmother of eight

Phone calls are really cheap – you buy these phone cards. I've got quite a bit of family abroad, but I speak to them four or five times a week. The oldest one doesn't talk as much now, because he's coming up to being a teenager. The girl probably talks the most and the youngest talks a bit. About a year ago, he went around the house with a cordless phone, asking me if I liked his new bedcover – he obviously thought it was like Skype and we could see him in his bedroom.

grandmother of five

There seems to be a common dislike of social networking as a means of keeping in touch:

I don't do Facebook. I can't be bothered and I don't want to know everything about everybody – it absolutely doesn't appeal. They've all got Facebook and things, so they tell me about theirs. And I find out about things that are happening from other parts of the family, because I've got a sister who's got six children and I see her once a week or so.

grandmother of one

I won't do Facebook or Twitter – they're so time-consuming and I don't like the way people lay out their inner souls on Facebook. It's opening yourself to a world that doesn't know you. Your most private things, you should be least proud of, you're throwing this out to the world – it's awful.

grandmother of eight

Views about using Skype are mixed:

My husband likes Skype and uses it quite a bit, but I'm less keen. If we Skype my son's family, they will sit there and the boys will drift past and drift away again. Whereas if you ring people up, you can speak to them directly. But with Skype you can say, 'Oh, you've had your hair cut' or 'That's a nice pair of pyjamas', so there are certainly advantages to it.

grandmother of ten

We call and we email. I found Skype too stressful and I didn't want to stress the children. My son told me that he used to have Skype appointments with them, but they wouldn't come to the screen and he'd get incredibly upset about it and then stopped. I'm very susceptible to them feeling stressed and also I don't like being rejected.

grandmother of three

One grandmother comments on the difficulty of being out of touch:

I went away for nine weeks last year and when I came back, so many things had changed. What I see with my friends with grandchildren abroad, is that if they don't see them for three or six months, the children have changed school or started ballet class and the grandparents need a crash course in what the children are up to.

Whereas by keeping regular contact, even if only for an hour or so, you can see the gradual development. And if there is something new in their life, they burst in going, 'Granny, I went to football, it's really good.'

grandmother of two

Chapter 4
The Emotional Side

Grandmothers clearly enjoy discussing the many things they do with their grandchildren. But the significance of being a grandmother does not arise solely from what they do, but equally from what they *feel*. This chapter explores the comments of grandmothers about the emotional side of their relationship with their grandchildren, from the inevitable love and pride to a lot of worrying.

Love and its expression
The principal emotion of any grandparent is a sense of love, often to a surprising degree. Grandmothers seek different ways to explain what this means:

> It really is like falling in love. You've got this all-encompassing, must-protect-at-all-costs feeling – a glow. It's wonderful. You've got to do everything you possibly can to make sure that nothing ever, ever happens to this person. It's almost as if you've got a double duty, because you don't want your child to be hurt or this child as well – you've got to work twice as hard.
>
> *grandmother of one*

> They teach you about love. They teach you about loving people for what they are – appreciating their individuality, their personalities, the tiny bits of other family members that you see coming through in them. You feel a terribly strong emotion.

> When the first granddaughter was born in Australia, we went to see her and spent six

months. I cried almost all the way home – it kept coming over me, that I was leaving this little child and I wouldn't see her again for a long while. I get more phlegmatic now, because I know that I'll be back, but it's still a sad thing to leave a wee one that you've got to know.

grandmother of ten

All grandchildren need is love. Not because they will do this or that for you, but because it's the right thing – it's something from you that's extended. You love your grandchildren as you love your own child. They don't all have the same character – some are difficult, some are easy – but you give them all love.

grandmother of three

Some describe this as a sense of kinship or having some special link:

There's an immediate kind of recognition – it's a look in the eye, it's a feeling of 'you and me understand each other'. I can't explain it, but there's definitely some sort of bond. You can feel it with a new baby.

I used to see a lot of one granddaughter when she was very young. She and I always get on well together, we have a kind of understanding. I don't know what it is – maybe we are quite alike, there's something we recognise in each other.

grandmother of eight

She was a lovely baby, very bright and always a joy to be with. I used to see her a lot. I still remember the first time she gave me a look of recognition. She was probably about three months old – we were in the park and it was getting quite cold and I remember putting my scarf over her pushchair and she just gave me a look, and I knew that she knew who I was. It was like a little *person*, kind of looking at me and saying, 'I know you – we know each other.'

grandmother of one

A few comment on their fear of not loving their grandchildren because they were already so much in love with their own children:

When the first grandchild was born, I was really worried because I thought, I love my daughter to pieces, and I'm never going to find enough love for a grandchild. I don't want to take any love from my daughter, she's my whole life. But the minute I saw this little bundle there, with a mat of black hair that looked exactly like my daughter did when she was born, I was in love again.

grandmother of two

You cannot believe that you would ever love anyone as much as you love your own children. But, you just do. When I was pregnant with my second child, I worried about that – how can I ever love anybody as much as I love my little boy? But they bring the love with them.

You have exactly the same feelings for the second one as you did the first, and I have the same feelings for my granddaughter as I did my two children. I just love her and I look forward to seeing her. It gives me great pleasure to see her happy.

grandmother of one

One argues that this love is all encompassing:

Having those grandkids – you don't need a man, you don't need a life, nothing else matters. That gives you everything! You don't need anything else in your life. That's how I felt for the first year. I still feel it now, but I was on a high for about a year.

grandmother of two

There is some disagreement about whether the love is different than the love for a woman's own child:

I tell everyone, it is just like being the mum. I've heard people say that it's a different kind of love to the love you have for your children. I don't know where they get that from. I love my grandson exactly the same as I love my kids – it's equal. You fall in love with your kids and it's just like having your own child all over again. The only difference is that you never had to go through the pain of childbirth.

grandmother of one

It's a completely different love to what you have for your own children. I don't know how to explain it, really, but you love them differently. Maybe you love them _more_. You love your children, obviously, but you haven't got all the work with the grandchildren. You haven't got all the hard things, you just get all the nice bits. So, when you have them, it's special.

grandmother of six

I'm not in the least bit maternal, never have
been. I'd never even held a baby until she was
put in my arms. My reaction to babies was
generally 'It's a baby, they throw up on you'.
When my grandson was born, it was
extraordinary – I probably felt more maternal
towards him then I did my children at first sight
– I just felt an instant link to him.

grandmother of two

And one grandmother compares it to the love for a
husband:

Some people love their husbands more than their
children. I never did. It's the just the love of a
man – he can go or I can go, but a daughter is for
life. That was my responsibility for the rest of
my life and nothing was ever going to harm her
if I could help it. It's the same with a grandchild.
I will walk over hot coals for my grandchildren
and my daughter. I can't believe that something
so wonderful happened to me because I don't
think I really deserved it.

grandmother of two

One talks about how she put her feelings into an
artistic form:

I made a pottery figure of me and him, at the
point he was learning to walk, and loved nothing
so much as to be held so that he could stand up.
For hours he wanted to be held. So, it's me,
grandmother, and him and it's called 'Uplift' –

I'm raising him up. It's also God and me and God's raising me up.

It comes from the beautiful feeling. They will come up and suddenly cuddle me and say 'I love you.' I feel quite tremble-y talking about it. It's 'I need you, I feel close to you' love. It's something about trust and security and closeness and unconditional love.

grandmother of two

In contrast, one great-grandmother describes how it is harder to be close when there are so many generations:

You try to be close with the great-grandchildren, but you never can be. You're back of the queue – there's the mum, then the grandmother, and then there's you. It's hurtful sometimes, because you want to be the same as you were with your grandchildren, but you can't take over the grandmother's part.

If I decide that I want to do something for my great-granddaughter, and her grandmother decides to do something, they're going to go with her. I'm older and I'm not in their league any more. I think they want to be with someone younger, that understands them more. And there's another set of great-grandparents as well.

grandmother of seven

Watching them grow
Although related to a general love, grandmothers also love the opportunity to watch their grandchildren grow and develop:

When I had my own children, I didn't notice them growing, because I was so busy. But just observing the grandchildren become their own selves is a miraculous experience. It's like seeing a little blob of nothing become a living creature right in front of you. They're all very civilised children, but I notice their aggression towards each other. When they start playing, the same thing happens with each child. It's like watching humanity develop in front of you.

grandmother of five

She's really clever – she learned to walk at ten months. You're teaching her things and it's lovely to see her grow and develop. You think she's been on this planet before because she's just so forward in what she does. To think how small she was, to see how she is now and look what she's doing. She's content, she's happy. It's just a lovely feeling.

grandmother of one

It's just lovely seeing them develop. I'm interested in everything they do. And, I always feel proud when they do well at things. My daughter phoned up and said her son got 'student of the week' – I felt genuinely pleased about that. You've just got other people to care about – you share their happy times and share when they're not so happy. I'm very grateful to have the time with them.

grandmother of five

Feeling connected

Grandmothers also talk about their general pleasure in having grandchildren in their lives:

> I tend to light up when I talk about my grandchildren. I just feel very connected to these expanding, joyful, alive little beings, who are so engaged with life and with me. And helping them to grow and find out and providing things that they enjoy and helping them – giving them the beginnings of wisdom. Just being close to them.
>
> *grandmother of two*

> It is wonderful having a young person again in your life, and because of the way we've always related, she's just been part of it all. She just is there, bright and bubbly, and lets me adore her. She's a teenage girl, sharing 'This is what's happening to me' – she wants me to know what's happening in her life.
>
> *grandmother of one*

> It's great just getting to know them as people. This is why I'm enjoying the little one so much more now – he's talking and he's starting to ask questions. It's just watching them develop and stretch themselves and find out about things. I've kind of learned to like children, which I never thought I would.
>
> *grandmother of two*

This may be particularly important when other parts of their life are not going well:

Grandchildren give you such pleasure. After my husband passed away, I was totally lost. And when they came into my life, all the time I was just thinking of them. My friends know this, they said, 'Look, you are very sad that you lost your husband, but God has created a situation for you which keeps you so busy – and look at you now. You talk of nothing but them, all the time.'

These grandchildren are my life. I would have been lost without them.

grandmother of four

Physical contact

Related to love is the pleasure of touch. Some grandmothers feel this is yet another source of deep enjoyment they obtain from grandchildren. It is particularly the case with babies:

All the kisses and the cuddles – lovely, can't beat it. That is the best bit of it. A lot of it comes from her mother's ways, because they kiss when they meet you and they kiss when they go. If I'm round her house, and her brothers and sisters come, they all kiss me – it's all a loving thing. I've started to change from being involved with her.

grandmother of eight

I'm very much like my mum in how I brought my kids up. Very loving, we could all get in bed with her. And all my kids could all get in bed with me. I have the grandkids in. Their mum doesn't allow that at home, but when they're with me, they get in. That's one rule that I broke and their mother knows. I love them next to me.

grandmother of six

When she was a baby, she would just let herself be cuddled. The wonder of a baby who allows you to love them, who lets you hold them, who is all flesh and wanting to be kissed, is wonderful. She would just sit there and allow herself to be loved.

She's becoming a tomboy now, but when I go to kiss her, she allows me, whereas her sister stays very stiff until you kiss her, and then goes away. This one is much freer with her soft body.

grandmother of five

One talks about the ache from the absence of touch, felt by her mother-in-law:

When I married my second husband, his mother was 83 – she had two grandsons but it was the first granddaughter, and she was thrilled. But she was too frail to hold the baby by herself, although she would've loved to. There was an immense sense of longing there. I used to take the baby down there, even though it's a long journey.

grandmother of two

Sometimes, the pleasure of touch comes particularly from the fact that it was initiated by the child:

I used to look after my little grandson when his mum was at work and after lunch, he would seem to be in a very happy space. I remember pushing him along in his pushchair and him reaching out his hand to me.

There was something very special about that little hand reaching for mine – not because he needed anything at that moment, he was as much giving me something back, giving me love. I wasn't expecting it – it wasn't 'I'll give you this and then you give me that', it was 'I will give you everything I can'. It was unconditional love. It was just beautiful.

grandmother of two

Touch is very important. Even today, my teenage granddaughter will come in, she will give you such a big hug and stand there hugging you. It really makes you feel so good. It makes you feel wanted, and loved. You can see that they don't do it for the sake of doing it, like just giving a quick kiss. They'll see me and their eyes shine.

Sometimes we arrive without telling them, they'll open the door and be so excited. My grandson will be on his computer, but he'll get up and come running and say, 'Oh, you've come!' They are not saying, 'Oh, God, these two oldies have arrived.'

grandmother of two

For those with family problems, this can be a very painful issue:

I try not to get too attached to the baby. I have done that once or twice – I allowed myself to feel and it was very painful when he didn't come for the next day or two. So I am playing with the remote control for my emotions, so that I don't

get that overwhelming feeling of wanting to hold
– and more, more, more.

My daughter called today and asked me to look
after him tomorrow night and I said to bring him
a bit earlier. I shouldn't have said that, I should
have asked her to bring him later, so that by the
time I feed him and put him in bed, it will be
enough. I need to keep that type of balance.

grandmother of one

One grandmother comments that some people have
become too suspicious of touch and children:

Children don't get enough physical contact these
days, partly because there's this suspicion of
physical contact. In the family, it's natural to
have physical contact. They were both climbing
over me last night – I was sitting on the floor
reading to them. And neither of them had a
stitch of clothing on.

grandmother of two

And one thinks touch has become too frequent in
modern culture:

My grandson hugs me more than I hug him. I
don't really like hugging. He'll come and sit on
my lap and kiss and hug me. My family and
friends laugh at me and say, 'Look! She's got a
grandson on her lap. He's made you do that,
hasn't he!'

I'm just not a tactile person. I see too much of it,
the young girls hugging and kissing when they
meet. It's so meaningless! I don't want to kiss

somebody that I don't even know. I'll just shake your hand, thank you. You can love in different ways.

grandmother of one

Talking about the grandchildren

One measure of the interest that grandmothers take in their grandchildren might be the extent to which they are eager to talk about them. Grandmothers are famous for pulling out their photos as soon as anyone expresses an interest or even before. This is also the case among many here:

First, there are the photographs:

I'm always ramming my photos in people's faces. They just say, 'Oh, he is gorgeous' or 'Doesn't he look like his mother?' No one's actually said I went on too much – my friends all ask me about him.

grandmother of one

We put loads of photos up of her on Facebook and, because my sister lives abroad, they're up for her to see – she says, 'She's lovely, isn't she getting big?' People must be thinking we're overwhelming them with all these photos, but we do it so people can see how she's progressing, how she's growing up.

grandmother of one

Then, there are the many stories of what the grandchildren are doing or discussions of how their own children don't get their child-rearing right:

I talk about my grandchildren a lot. I tell friends how they're getting on, what they've been doing in school – I'm proud of them. Two of them have applied to be on the X-Factor and I'll say if they're going to be going on that. I don't overdo it, because I know it can be boring.

grandmother of seven

At work, we all talk about our grandchildren – things like disagreeing about how the parents do things come up all the time. It seems like it's a normal part of being a grandparent, how you look at what the parents are doing and say, 'I wouldn't do that.'

grandmother of two

But quite a few are anxious to distance themselves from such a practice. This is partly because they see it as likely to be annoying to other people:

I don't carry photos. I think it is boring for other people. And I don't tell people all the time what my grandchildren are doing. If other grandmothers show me theirs, I look at their photos, and say, 'Oh, how lovely.' But you don't generally want to hear what someone else's grandchildren are eating and what they've said and I don't tell other people about mine. You have to be a little sensitive that not everybody's grandchildren are doing exactly the same.

grandmother of eleven

I can remember being somewhere before I was a grandmother – there were three or four people going on about their grandchildren and handing photos round. I found it hard to take. I know someone who's lost her grown-up children, who certainly wouldn't want to know about families. And there are others who might be wanting to be a grandmother and not knowing if it's going to happen. I don't want to be a bore.

grandmother of two

But it is also because they feel that their feelings are a private matter:

I don't even start talking about my grandson. I think it's just so inappropriate and silly. Nobody can truly share the joy of having a grandchild. And talking about it in order to show importance is a futile exercise. Even if people say, 'Oh, he's a lovely cutie' or whatever, it's not defining my true feeling towards my grandson. I don't like others telling me how lovely my grandson is – I know how lovely he is. I think it's very private.

grandmother of one

I don't talk much about my private life at all. What's happening at the moment is just as interesting – the way the sun's shining, there's a robin in the garden, and have you read about so-and-so today? It doesn't take second place, but it is a part of a much bigger picture.

I've got photographs of them, of course, but everybody has their grandchildren. My grandchildren are not their grandchildren and why should they want to know?

grandmother of eight

And one recounts technical difficulties:

I don't share photos, because I don't know the technology. I took photographs of my daughters from the day they were born right up until they got married. But when they changed to the mobile phones and all that and you can't go and print them, I just stopped taking photographs. I keep telling them, give me your photographs, let me put them in an album, but they don't get round to it. I'm going on a course now to learn how to use the iPad.

grandmother of one

One grandmother has another view on the issue:

People turn up with their iPads covered in photos of the kids and they ask if I have any photos of my grandchildren – I say vaguely, 'Yes, somewhere.' I get turned off by people constantly seeing their lives through the lens of a camera. When my children were small, we couldn't afford a camera and I regret that I haven't got many photos, but in the long run it's not important because it's in your heart and in your head.

grandmother of two

In the occasional case, *not* talking about grandchildren is a deliberate policy among friends:

When I go out with my friends, we have make a pact that we're not going to talk about them or get any photos out. It's our night, a girls night out for five of us. Otherwise, we're all showing one another photos and we're showing the videos.

So we just go out and have a bottle of wine or a meal – have a chat like adults, *without* talking about the kids. But it's hard. You'll be chatting about something, what you did that day, and one of the grandkids will slip into the conversation.

grandmother of six

Worrying

Another sign of love is worrying. Grandmothers do a lot of this. Some of it is general worrying about all the possible things that might go wrong:

I got too involved at first. I used to worry are they eating? are they doing the right thing? are they getting up in the night? are they doing it all different to how I'd done it? – I was almost in a panic. It was *their* way, not my way, and I found that quite difficult.

grandmother of two

I worry about mugging, I worry about them coming home alone on the train. I tell him to put a £10 note in his shoes, because they can get mugged in the train. He listens. I said, 'I can't go with you everywhere, you have to learn to be adult, but you have to be streetwise.' If you don't tell them, how do they know? How are they going to get aware?

grandmother of two

A lot of the time, I feel anxious for everybody concerned. I think are they going to cope? How's it going to go? What can I do? Why aren't I doing more?' There's quite a lot of 'Why aren't I doing more?' in my life. Every time I think it through, I realise that I am probably doing as much as I can, but it's never enough.

As a parent or as a grandparent, you're never able to do enough. You want everything to be absolutely okay for everybody and you can't. My big catchphrase is 'Be there' – for all of them. If anybody ever wants me to do anything, I'm there. And if they don't, I won't push myself.

grandmother of eight

The possibility that grandchildren will get into drugs is a common cause of concern:

I cannot say my children or grandchildren haven't done drugs. I haven't seen them, so I don't know. But, I keep telling them if they get mixed up with anything like that, I'll stick with you all the way, but if you go and do anything that's wrong, don't come and call me because I won't be coming. I made it very clear.

grandmother of ten

As they get older, you have to be careful about finding out too much. As soon as I know they're going out, I think, Oh, my goodness, they must do this, they must do that. And then I think, Stop it, they're adults – you need to stand back. It's pointless becoming too anxious about it. My daughter did drugs as an older teenager. And there's nothing you can do about it anyway. The most you can say, is just be sensible and when she was older, just don't tell me about it. I don't actually want to know.

grandmother of one

You have all these street gangs. Children do things just to feel they are one of them. If you let them go with every Tom, Dick, and Harry, you don't know what they'll do – they ask friends to hand onto drugs for them and the next thing you know the police come. When my grandson started making friends, he started being 'cool'.

One has to be guiding one's children and grandchildren, protecting them. I try not to worry, but I worry for everybody.

grandmother of three

When grandchildren have reached adulthood, some worrying can be mutual:

They check on me all the time to see if I'm home, if they know I'm out late on my own. I no sooner get in then they're, 'Are you home, Grandma?' I do the same with them. If I know they're going to clubs, I say, 'Just phone me when you get home. I don't care if it's 3 or 4 in the morning.' I just want to know they're safely home. I worry that they'll get in a taxi and get attacked or somebody gives them a rape drug or those sort of things.

grandmother of two

And some worrying arises from very particular circumstances:

I worry about my daughter's kids because she's separated now and my son-in-law doesn't seem to contact the kids very often, so I worry that he might just drift out of their lives. I just hope they'll make good choices – in friends, in lifestyle, in education.

grandmother of five

There was a time when my teenage granddaughter disappeared – she was actually at a friend's house – but nobody knew where she was for one evening. It was all perfectly fine in the end. There were rules, you either came home or you phoned, you let somebody know, but the phone didn't work. I think she just couldn't be bothered.

Kids do that. I was frightened that something had happened to her – that she'd got run over, anything could've happened. But she's not any more thoughtless and ridiculous than any other teenager – or that we've all been.

grandmother of one

Grandchildren with problems or vulnerabilities are a particular source of worry. Some of this concerns the here and now:

When one granddaughter was little, I said it sounds like she might have dyslexia – get her checked – and three years later, they learned that she does have it. When she was only six years old, she came in and broke down: 'Nobody likes me, my friend hates me.' She's in here sobbing her heart out. It just got to me.

It turned out that the school has picked up on her dyslexia and she's getting extra help, but it segregates her. So she was feeling pressured with everything and everyone. At six years old, that's a hell of a lot.

grandmother of two

My grandson's always been very attached to his mother – emotionally, he hasn't really grown up. I think he's very bright, but not the conventional kind of intelligence and he is struggling immensely at school. I do get worried about that. I would like him to get the basic skills, but primary state schools don't really push children.

grandmother of three

But often it is about their longer term future:

We've spent a lot of time with one grandson, who's autistic, and we get on well with him. He has special needs and we understand those. He's quite high-functioning and a lovely person. I do worry about him. It's okay while he's at school, but it's that bit when he leaves school that I worry about. How will he be occupied? He struggles with personal relationships, but also in getting a meaningful occupation. So, yes, it's a worry.

grandmother of ten

I worry about my eldest grandson, because he's very highly strung and very fragile. We have schizophrenia in the family. I say to my daughter to be careful with him. I feel very protective, because he's had several meltdowns recently. He's just completely gone to pieces because the pressure at school is too much, and he loses all perspective. It's the teenage years when it really kicks in – he could also develop schizophrenia and mental health problems, because there is so much in my family.

grandmother of three

One of my granddaughters became badly brain damaged at the age of two and a half with a rare condition that the hospital didn't recognise. She can't talk or do anything for herself, even today, and she's an adult. But she does understand quite a lot and we really get on. She went to a special school.

They put on a play and all the children were wheeled round in their wheelchairs to do their part – she was on stage when she caught sight of me in the audience, her face went all red with effort and she called out to me by name! I've never forgotten that, because it's all tucked away in her mind there.

I find myself being anxious about what will happen to her. She's living at home, she's living a very good life. What happens if they can't look after her any longer? I can't talk to them about that, because they're adults and they wouldn't like it and they have lots of friends and they *must've* thought about it themselves.

grandmother of eight

The same grandmother also talks about her grandson who died of the same disease:

A year or so after the girl came home, her brother became ill. He was all right until then. He was rushed off to hospital, but he died very quickly. When he died, my feeling was a terrible helplessness that I couldn't help my daughter. I felt I was carrying it all for her. We all used to go and help her and talk to my granddaughter.

I think about him quite a lot. He's buried in a local graveyard and once a year, I pop in and leave some flowers for him. And of course it wasn't nearly as bad for me as it was for his parents. You can't imagine anything more awful happening, but somehow it was more awful than I thought it might be. I did seem to be carrying this burden for everybody. I still feel it to an extent.

grandmother of eight

Happy memories

And, of course, love also comes out in happy memories. These start with babies and toddlers:

I captured a very happy one moment when my baby grandson stood up for the first time, pushed a coffee table and drove it to a corner, and when there was no more space to go, he stood there and made the funniest noise. He looked at me, and I thought, are you challenging me to say the same as you? And I did – and we both laughed. That was absolutely the most beautiful thing that ever has happened so far. It was a mutual contact on a very happy level.

grandmother of one

I took one grandchild to a dance at the village hall, when she was two or three – just able to totter around. My neighbour was a folk guitarist and his group were playing – and we danced until 12 o'clock, she never got tired! And at her parent's wedding – they got married after she was born – it was the same thing, she just loved dancing. We danced together for hours and hours. That was great.

grandmother of eight

My happiest memory of them is me lying on the floor in my house, and they're walking all over me. They were toddlers just jumping on me. And when they finished, I was so sore where they jumped on me, but it was nice. I often think about that.

grandmother of ten

But some include somewhat older children:

We often go to a soft play centre – it's is a sort of a huge gymnasium, with lots of soft padding, so you can jump around, and a sunken trampoline, where all the adults can play as well. My daughter put together a 12-foot trampoline, and they said, 'Granny, you've got to have a go.' They got me on it, and they thought that was hilarious.

grandmother of three

They stay with me a lot and like to sleep with me. I love it. When they are lying in bed with me in the morning – that's the happiest time. We'll talk about anything, what should we do, what we are having for breakfast.

But what makes me so happy is that they are sharing their time with me. One is lying on my leg, one is lying on my hair, one is putting the fingers on my head – it's like a joyful current going all in my body. You can't buy that happiness anywhere.

grandmother of four

Sometimes, these centre around a holiday together:

I rented a flat and took them to Paris last year and they were wonderful. They liked the Louvre and the Eiffel Tower, of course. We stopped in a café and we spent about two hours just sitting and looking at people – that was a really nice time.

My granddaughter said that she wanted to cook something – she found a recipe on the internet and wrote a shopping list. We had found a little market, so we went shopping, and in the evening, she told me she didn't want me in the kitchen because she was doing the cooking. She did something really nice. She was trying to give me a treat – and that's what she did. It was wonderful.

grandmother of two

Last year, I took my daughter and her boys to France. They had a mobile home and I slept in my camper and we had a fortnight together – it was wonderful. The whole time we were in there was not adult time. We said it's not for us, it's for the boys, we'll do what will make them happy. We were on a campsite with a big swimming pool with slides in it, hundreds of other kids around, beach, hired bikes. We more or less went to bed when they did and got up when they did.

Just sitting outside the caravan, peeling some vegetables, watching those boys go up and down on scooters – it was great. Particularly the little two-year-old, who was completely naked apart from a pair of Wellingtons. And just seeing them in sunshine. The kids got up in the morning and didn't put clothes on – can we go in the swimming pool now? Just the enthusiasm – they absolutely loved it. It was just such a nice thing to do for them.

grandmother of two

Favourites and not so favourites

Most grandmothers feel that it is inappropriate to have any kind of favouritism and many say that it is not part of their thinking:

I determined to treat my two grandchildren equally. I might feel more strongly for one or the other, but I must be equally loving to them. That came from my parenting, because the sun shone out of my brother's backside. He'd get whatever he wanted from our mother. If he wanted it, he had it, even if it had been promised to me first. I felt undervalued. So treating equally is very strong.

grandmother of two

I never felt that I had favourites of my own children. And I don't feel that I have favourites with the grandchildren. They might tell you differently, but I don't think I have. Each one is so much its own personality, you adapt to that, really.

grandmother of eight

Nonetheless, the occasional grandmother suggests that it is difficult not to do so:

You shouldn't say it, but I would say one grandson is my favourite. Maybe because he's my first boy grandchild and I looked after him for a while. Although I love them all dearly, he and I were very close. He used to stay with me a lot too, just me and him. He reminded me very much of my son – he looks like him and has his character. Very loving.

grandmother of six

I love all my grandkids, but there's something special about one boy. When they went on holiday, and took him out of the country, I felt so upset. I had a lump in my throat, and I thought, why am I feeling like this? It was the thought that I couldn't go round the corner and see him. I told his mother how I felt and she said I shouldn't be silly, but I couldn't help it. I would never show that with any of them, whatever I felt.

grandmother of eight

And one grandmother talks about relationships differing due to personality:

It's a two-way thing, it's not just what *you* feel. The personality of the child dictates the relationship very much. You have to accept that, like with your own children, you aim to be equal, but you will have a different relationship with each of your grandchildren and some will be closer than others.

It's not to do with proximity. It's to do with the personality and character of the child – it's to do, literally, with the people that they are. Some are very open and loving and want to talk. Others are much more self-contained and they just don't. You definitely have to work harder with some.

grandmother of ten

One great-grandmother notes that those she sees are different simply because of that contact:

The great-grandchildren I see would be my favourites, because I see them. The ones that I don't see, I don't know, really. I still love them. When they come round I make a fuss over them, but I don't know them children as much as the ones that are around me.

grandmother of seven

The other side of the coin are the grandchildren that are liked less. This is even more of an uneasy subject. In fact, the difficulties experienced are of very different orders:

One grandson was a nightmare. He took money out of my purse when he was about 14. By all accounts, his mother was having problems with him, and she obviously got in touch with my son, the father, who brought him here and asked if he could stay. I said yes, as long as he behaves. But he was stealing out of my purse all the time. I knew, because nobody else ever did. And I just told my son he would have to take him away. His own mother said she had to lock everything away.

grandmother of eight

I struggle with one granddaughter, because she's got some mental health issues. Some doctors say she's got ADHD, others say she's got Asperger's, but I think she's probably just very naughty. I struggle with her naughtiness because I do love her. I can feel very hurt and almost hate her sometimes.

But I have also seen her be perfect – not stepping out of line, not saying anything rude to me or anything. My son's been to see different people and I think we might be on the right track now.

grandmother of five

I dislike my younger granddaughter – she's very spoilt and my daughter's kept the cute thing going, where she carries a blanket around, and I find it all very tedious. I've got more energy for the older one, because I can see he's fragile, he's intelligent, and he's desperate for someone to give him a bit of attention.

grandmother of three

Some simply don't like certain stages:

I didn't like my grandson when he was a little baby. I don't like caring for little babies – their nappies, the crying. I didn't change the nappies. I just said to my daughter, 'You're the mum, you have to bond with your baby – you change his nappy, you bathe him.' I love him now that he can talk.

grandmother of one

Those with little or no access to their grandchildren
The emotional side of relationships with grandchildren would not be complete without some discussion of the less happy stories. It is easy to talk about the love, even when it is coupled with worry. It is much less easy to talk about where there is little or no access to their grandchildren.

Some lose contact altogether:

> I don't have any dealings with my daughter. I don't see her children. It hurt at first. Although I fell out with her, she said that I could still see the boys, but I would have to come and get them. I think she wanted me to still have contact with *her*, which I didn't want. And I thought, if they want to see me when they're older, they will.

> She's just not a nice person. She was really slagging me off to people. I don't know what her problem was. When she was grown up, I did so much for her, picking up her kids from the nursery, taking her to work if she had an evening job and picking her up. None of it was appreciated. She would say 'Oh, you don't do anything for me.' and I would think to myself, you've got a very short memory. I can't say I miss her, because I don't.
> *grandmother of eight*

And some have so little contact that it feels a very distant relationship:

> My daughter married someone from a different culture, and had a baby here. They went to live abroad, but they moved back a year ago. In that

time, I've been round to their house very little –
I'm just not welcome there. Her husband doesn't
like any visitors at all – none of her friends,
nothing. Even when she might visit me, he'd say,
'Leave the baby at home, go and see your mum
on your own.'

I've probably seen the baby three times. It's
very hard. I won't say anything to my daughter,
because it puts her in a difficult position – it's
her husband, you can't really do that.

It's a bit strange, because my little granddaughter
doesn't know me at all. She's probably sees me as
just another adult. She goes to nursery and is used
to mixing with adults. The father's quite happy to
send her to a nursery, run by strangers who don't
have the same belief system or any of the same
background, but doesn't want to bring her here.
My daughter says it wouldn't be any different if I
lived around the corner. So what can you do?

grandmother of one

One of my sons has been very successful. He's a
builder and he's built lots of houses and he's got
a place in Spain. He's worked hard for what he's
done, but I feel he's big-headed and looks down
on some of them. I get annoyed and tell him not
to forget where he's come from. I don't actually
see a lot of his children. When they come, they
kiss me and say they love me, but I've not been
in their life a lot.

grandmother of seven

Others have strained relationships within the family
and therefore miss out on seeing their grandchildren as

much as they would like or in as easy a way as they would like:

> If my daughter is in charge of her children for the next two weeks, I know I am going to see less of them. They come at 7 o'clock – 'Sorry, no time, they have to go to bed.' So, I'm seeing less of my grandchildren now.
>
> Whereas if her brother is in charge of them – they take turns looking after the children – he's going to bring them to me and make a point of my enjoying them. He knows what pleasure it gives me. She doesn't care if it gives me pleasure or not, she's got to be doing the right thing towards her children in the right way.
>
> *grandmother of five*

> The baby was crying a lot when he was very small. I went to the health food shop and got a special tea for colic pain. I took this to my daughter's place and was reading the instructions when her husband said I mustn't give anything to the baby – 'Either you leave now or I'm going to take him upstairs and lock us in a room so you cannot reach him.' He said I shouldn't come back ever until I was invited.
>
> I got very angry but said nothing and left. I drove a little bit past the house and then I stopped and cried and cried. I went back the next day. My bond with my daughter is greater than a fool's behaviour. I just ignored him. But I think I have a missed a lot, being expelled, pushed out.
>
> *grandmother of two*

Access has been used as a threat sometimes. My son-in-law will say, 'You won't see them' and so on, but my daughter always says, 'Forget it, that will *never* happen.' It's very difficult. He has sometimes left here slamming the door and taking the kids and I wasn't too sure when I was going to see them again.

I know he feels sorry after, but it's a kind of pattern. And every time it hurts. It's getting better now. I can see when he's getting into that frame of mind and I try to detach myself, because I would rather not go through any confrontation. I know I'll see them on my own again and we will get on fine.

grandmother of three

And there are those who have access, but feel they are constantly constrained, wanting to do much more:

My daughter hardly ever asked if we could come and look after the first child. He was about two and a half before we were invited to do so, even for a couple of hours. Now, if we are there, it sometimes happens that we entertain the children while my daughter does some emailing or whatever. But we'd love to give them more – just do little things, such as taking them out to the local park. All of my friends seem to be much more involved in raising their grandchildren.

They're lovely children and we see them, so we can't grumble, but I feel quite excluded. It isn't a thing I can discuss with my daughter, other than to make endless offers – 'Why don't you go out to the cinema or a meal, we'll come and babysit? She always says 'Oh, I don't think we're ready for that.' I don't want to set up any kind of conflict between them, because life is hard enough when you're young parents. We just live with it. I don't think it's ever going to change.

grandmother of two

Individual grandchildren
It was clear from the beginning that this book is about grandmothers – not their grandchildren. But in the course of discussions, some grandchildren seemed to creep in and become personalities demanding attention. Here are a small number, of differing ages:

One little one loves to phone us. He learned our phone number when he was only three and he rings every morning! Sometimes, that's at 7.00 a.m. – fortunately we're early risers. He once rang us up at 6.00 a.m. and that was a little early. He doesn't ask, he just gets the phone and thinks he'll have a chat.

He tells us all sorts of things. He'll tell us his mother and father are in bed asleep, and I know they're not, because they leave the house early. He just likes to get on the phone and chat. So, when the phone rings in the morning, I know it's him.

grandmother of eleven

My 17 year old grandson is handsome, bright and very introverted. He plays the organ in a church on a Sunday morning. I go and feel so proud. There are all these elderly ladies and they dote on him, because he's a young lad. They'll give him a kiss and say, 'Oh, our service is going to be so good.' They come to me and they say, 'Your son is doing very well' and I say, 'No, he's my grandson.'

The day that the GCSE results were coming, I rang up early in the morning, asking my daughter about the results, because they're posted at midnight, so I expected him to stay up to see them. No, he went to bed. And he wouldn't tell them his password, so they waited until 7.00 in the morning, and pressed him to look into it and he said, 'Not now, Dad, I'm sleeping.' At 8 o'clock, I rang up and his mum took the phone to his room. I said, 'I want to know now – the suspense, I'm dying!' Do you want to come home and see a dead Nani?' So, they put the phone on speaker, and he counted one by one and eventually there were eleven A*s. We took him out for a celebration.

grandmother of two

My granddaughter was always very quiet, very serious. And you felt she was judging you, even at age two or three. When she looked at me, I felt she knew much more about me than she was saying, like an old person's soul in her little face. I wished I could hide. She's very intuitive and very bright. She's at university now, studying to be a psychologist. She's sultry and sophisticated and she's grown into herself. She's quite stunning.

grandmother of two

One grandson is 19. He ducks and dives. His father was a car dealer and he's quite the same.

He's in and out all the time, six times a day. In the fridge, gets a drink, whatever, 'You all right, Nan?' and then he's gone. He'll come back and he'll go straight in the loo. He'll often come in here and give me a kiss and I know he wants something. And then it's 'Nan, can I borrow your car for a minute?'

You cannot tell him anything, he knows better. I say, 'I'm 70 and you're 19, and you know better than me?' And he laughs. I do try to steer him, but they will do what they want to do. You can't pin him down.

He used to live here. I slung him out because he was so rude. I said, 'My kids have never done that – out! Don't come back.' I didn't speak to him for quite a few years. He was living at his other nan's. He asked if he could come back and I said, 'No – you only get one chance with me.' You've got to draw a line. The other nan doesn't want him there, but she won't sling him out. But we slowly got back to seeing each other. I was sitting outside in the summer with a neighbour, having a drink of an evening. He came along and said, 'All right, Nan?' and I went, 'All right.' And that was it – he was in the garden, and back in my house.

I love him to bits. I just don't like the person he is. I'll always love him, but I wouldn't have him back. My son says he'll grow out of it, but I don't know. He talks to me quite nicely, now. He daren't not, because he won't get his foot over the doorstep if he back-chats me. It's so disrespectful.

grandmother of eight

105

I have quite a special relationship with one grandson, who is now in his twenties. My son married on the rebound and had him straight away. They split up and, at one stage, when the boy was 8 or 9, she moved away and just disappeared off the face of the earth. I felt awful. I just felt bereft – on my son's behalf, as much as on mine.

I always liked this grandson. We got on quite well and I saw him fairly often early on. Then for three or four years, we didn't know where he'd gone. During that time, my son was offered a job abroad. If the boy had been around, he wouldn't have taken it, but he did and they lost touch. When the boy was 12, he phoned me and asked if I knew where his dad was. We met up and I took him to see his father. When I brought him back, he'd spent all his money on a beautiful scarf for his mother and she wasn't interested. So, all of that was terribly hard. It was heart-rending.

We have a very close relationship now. I have kind-of stood in for his father. He is still trying to be like his father and show him who he is. He's at university now and he's doing very well. He's married, has a little girl, but his wife has had post-natal depression. He really has shouldered everything, while being extremely badly off.

But she is getting help and they are hoping that she will be able to go back to work eventually. In the meantime, my great-granddaughter goes to nursery and she's very bright. I don't see them as often as I'd like, but we keep in touch by email. I usually go down there and we have lunch together and go for a walk by the sea.

grandmother of eight

Chapter 5
Views on Child-Rearing

Being a grandmother almost always means watching how the children bring up their children. Grandmothers cannot help but notice and often have strong opinions. This can be the source of great pleasure, but it can also be a difficult issue on both sides. This chapter explores some of the complexities here.

Parental approval

It is the lucky grandmother who is wholly approving of the child-rearing of their children, but many do exist. Not only are they very positive, but they feel their children are doing much better than they did:

> I'm hugely admiring of her ability to have the energy and the resources to do the things she needs to do, like instil the right level of discipline and support, draw the boundaries clearly and make sure the children are loved. If they don't do what they're supposed to do, both parents are extremely firm, they back each other up. When it was me, dragging my kids up, I just ran out of steam.
>
> ### *grandmother of two*

> I always thought she was a better mother – that's manifested in their very close relationship. I'm pretty sure they talk about everything, whereas my daughter and I do talk about everything now, but it was not so much when she was a teenager.
>
> ### *grandmother of one*

This provides an opportunity to muse on the long-term effects of their own child-rearing:

They listen well as parents. I was too busy. We had to run a very regimented house to allow everything to run smoothly. But my kids feel they had a happy childhood. And that's, perhaps, the most important thing – I hope their children feel the same. It's all you can give your children, really, is a happy childhood and happy memories.

grandmother of eleven

One mother comments with approval of her son and his partner's careful management of a complete separation and its effect for her granddaughter:

My granddaughter knew what was going on when they separated. Credit to them, they really negotiated that extremely well and there was no volatility. They lived ten minutes away from each other and remained parenting alongside each other very actively. My son was excellent in supporting her as a friend and co-parent, and making sure that his daughter was provided for.

I was hugely relieved that they were so communicative with each other, having known the opposite with the father of my children. So I really respected them enormously and admired them.

grandmother of three

Disagreements on child-rearing

But, of course, there are also many who note problems with the upbringing of their grandchildren. Many of these are relatively minor problems.

Material things

Perhaps the most common complaint concerns the amount of things their grandchildren have:

> Sometimes I say that I think they have too much, too many material things. I tell the grandchildren that too. They often laugh – they know that Grandma just doesn't understand life today. When I had my children, we would discuss whether they *needed* something, not just getting it because they wanted it.
>
> **grandmother of eleven**

> I think they have too much – toys and stuff. In my day, you just had maybe a couple of toys. Their house is like one big playroom. He can't play with everything. You couldn't move for the stuff under my Christmas tree – and half of it she would find six months later, not even out of the wrapping. In fact, we found an old hair dryer and that's what that child plays with all the time. So, all these toys, I just think, why?
>
> **grandmother of eight**

> They all have far too much stuff. All my friends say that about their grandchildren. It's just ridiculous. I don't even give them toys anymore. I told my grandson, when it was his birthday, that I would only give them *experience* presents now, like taking them to the theatre.
>
> **grandmother of five**

The use of time

As children grow older, television and computer games are another big issue:

One thing I find difficult is the way the huge screen television was on all the time in the living room – at meals, the girls would slip out to watch telly. I think it's a pity if that's allowed to happen.

grandmother of eight

The real tension is around screen time – iPhone, iPad, Minecraft and all this stuff they have. We took them abroad to a nice resort, and they just wanted to stay in their room and have screen time. It's almost like an addiction. You ask them to stop, 'But I have to get to the end of this game.' or 'I've got to get to the next level.' Everybody I know with kids of this age finds it's a huge problem.

grandmother of five

He wanted an X-Box for Christmas and of course he wasn't getting one, but he's got a DS, one of these little games. If I need to take the dog out, I'll ask him 'Fancy coming into my world?' and he'll tell me he just got onto another level. Once you get him out, he's fine, but they do get hooked.

grandmother of two

The issue is not simply about what the grandchildren are doing, but also about what activities they are then missing out on:

A lot of young parents are not talking to their children. There's too much reliance on the television and less *doing* things with them. I'd like to teach young people about how you should interact with children, but there's so much resistance. It's so much easier to bring them up the way they're doing it.

People say that when many children go to school, they can't talk, they can't communicate, they don't understand a lot of things. So all those wonderful years for the children to become so solid and beautiful, you're wasting them in not talking to them! With my grandson, I'm practising what I feel.

grandmother of one

We found an old Scrabble set and I was teaching the nine-year-old how to play. I realised that, in between turns, he was playing games on his mini-iPad. His mother came in and got very cross, telling him he was being rude, and he said 'Well, it is a boring game, isn't it?' My sister told me that she *made* her kids play cards and they had a good time.

grandmother of five

Other issues
There are also other matters that can arise. Manners can be a source of annoyance to the older generation:

I just can't stand it when they eat like pigs at the table. Whenever the kids come down to visit, I think they must've had a big talking-to about manners beforehand. Once, when the parents were both at work, I asked the kids if they had finished their tea, and the little one said, 'Thank-you-very-much-for-my-tea-it-was-very-nice-and-please-may-I-now-leave-the-table.' He said it all like he'd been practising it for about two weeks.

grandmother of five

Strictness about food is another source of conflict:

There are so many things the parents do in a different way. Like food. In my view, your child doesn't like this thing, fine, give him something different. But my son-in-law is strict – he'll let them have only what is good for them, and thinks if we don't tell them now, they'll never learn.

I'm not in favour of forcing them to do this or do that and having the tears in the eyes. As they grow up a little bit more, slowly, slowly, you teach them and they will learn.

grandmother of four

Some grandmothers are concerned about too much hygiene, albeit for different reasons:

My daughter has lots of rules and regulations and she's really *fussy* about hygiene. I'm not a dirty person, but she wants everything meticulous, too clean – one little dot and she wants to change the baby! They want to wash the towels every day. It creates a lot of work.

grandmother of two

They are very fastidious about being clean. I do worry a bit, when I read reports about modern children being allergic to everything, because they're not exposed to enough dirt. I was raised in a medical family. My father said the dirtiest families in his practice were often the ones that had nothing wrong with them, whereas those who were clean went down with everything.

grandmother of two

Disagreements about child-rearing can be particularly difficult where the mother and grandmother live together, as noted by one great-grandmother:

> My daughter's the mother, of course, but if I don't like what she's saying, I will say something. Like her son, I don't want him bringing girls back home all the time. I didn't allow my children to do that. I wouldn't like some boy to be doing that to my daughter or granddaughter. If I think they're being overly rude to their mum, I will speak to them.
>
> ***grandmother of seven***

Larger problems

All of these issues are annoying, but they are not fundamental to the way a child is brought up. A few grandmothers note more worrying problems:

> My son can be so strict – there's no place for discussion, they have to listen, even when there is absolutely no need for a Sergeant Major approach. I find that difficult. I won't intervene because he would get really angry. He'd say that it's not my place to say anything and he can bring up his children the way he wants and so on – it's a bit upsetting.
>
> ***grandmother of three***

> My daughter would love her children to be high achievers, but she has realised that her son is not as bright as she thinks. She's disappointed by it and the child feels it and wants to do the best for his mother. He doesn't want to do his homework, but he says he has to.

I tell him to relax a bit, and he says 'No, I *have* to!' It's torture to watch him. He's had lessons in Kumon, he's had lessons in French – he's had lessons pushed down his throat because his mother wants him to be a high achiever.

grandmother of five

One grandmother describes the inability of her son, with major problems of his own, to care for his twins:

One time, we were in a café and he had the twins on his own –and they were wild. They were flinging off their snowsuits and boots going everywhere and we're in a place trying to eat some pasta and it's like 'Oh, my God!' Very difficult. With twins, they're a unit – they know how to challenge, and they do it at the same time.

I didn't think he could handle them and I was worried about their safety. He told me he couldn't. He would sometimes ring me and say, 'I'm freaking out, I don't know what to do.' He would be off his head on something and not paying attention. It was horrible.

grandmother of three

Offering advice
Both mothers and mothers-in-law are famous for trying to advise parents on their children's upbringing. Sometimes, this is thought to be very welcome:

I didn't want to be one of those grandmothers where she'll get annoyed with me, and say, 'He's *mine*, not yours.' I used to tell her to let me know if she felt I was trying to take over. But she said I'd brought up three of my own and she loved my advice. Never once did she say, 'Mum, you're getting on my nerves,' because she knew that what I was telling her was for the best. Now she says she couldn't have done it without me.

grandmother of one

I'm quite easy-going and I realise that people have to make their own mistakes. They've both done things when I've thought, oh, that won't work, but you let them get on with it. I've got a good relationship with them and they do ask me what I think, like bedtime routines, or problems with weaning.

If they have any kind of problem, they usually ring me immediately – even now. I'm extremely lucky, because a lot of people don't have that with their kids.

grandmother of three

But grandmothers are well aware that their advice may not be appreciated and some do their best not to interfere:

Every grandmother has to be issued with a zip. There's a fine line between help and interference and you have to learn it. Nobody can teach it to you, because everybody's experience is different.

My mother-in-law was always so busy trying not to interfere that she wasn't actually much help. I used to say to my husband that we could do this or that if his parents would just have the children for two hours, but he didn't like to ask. We used to have to say, 'Shall we come over? Would you like to see them?'

grandmother of two

One of the interesting things about being a grandmother is that you would like to get your ideas across without them feeling you're criticising them. There's no point in putting their backs up, because then you won't see them at all and you won't have any chance to do anything.

I haven't interfered. If I had, my daughter might have got very cross with me, and my son-in-law just might not have wanted the mother-in-law around. I've got a strong personality and quite strong views about things, but it is *not* my role to impress those onto other people and the way they live.

grandmother of eight

You have to support the parents. If the parent says they are not to do something, then generally speaking, you should support that. Sometimes you have to be silent. There are times, particularly with the teenage girls, who are naturally rebelling where you don't always agree with the parents' attitude. That can be a bit hard – they've got their own reasons, but it's not the way you would've done it.

grandmother of ten

There's an unspoken, tacit contract that you absolutely don't undermine the authority of the parent. I don't want that authority, that responsibility. I want to be able to walk away. I want to know that the parents are absolutely in control here. And they need the confidence to be able to carry on doing that.

grandmother of two

Much of the time, grandmothers tip-toe around the issues, trying to find the most sensitive way of expressing their concerns:

You make suggestions. When the baby wasn't sleeping, you'd say, 'Well, is she warm enough? Does she have a bottle before she goes to bed?' and things like that. You just try to make their life a little bit easier, but at the same time, they make their own decisions. I think that is important.

grandmother of one

I decided very early on that I'd only say something if I felt that what they were doing was actually damaging. If it was different from the way I'd do it, then I might say, 'I used to do it this way,' but I'm unlikely to say anything. My daughter-in-law made it clear that she wanted me to grandparent in the way that felt right to me. I thought it was very good that she said that.

grandmother of two

My daughter's not always easy, and I would say, 'Is it okay if I do this? Because when I had you, I did this, but I know that I haven't read all the books and you have.' These 30-something mothers, they have a whole library of books, how to get your baby to sleep, and don't do this, and do do that. For me, you just pick them up and feed them. I was working, you just get on with it.

grandmother of two

And sometimes, not saying something is also effective:

I don't interfere, because I don't want them to hate me. I'm not a talker. I think it hurts them more when I *don't* talk, because they don't know what I'm thinking. When I go quiet, they know to keep away.

grandmother of ten

Occasionally, a grandmother will intervene more forcefully, rather than simply offering advice:

After the second one was born, I got quite worried for them. I can remember inviting myself over at tea time, because that was the worst time for my daughter. She wanted to spend time with the older one, but when you've got this screaming baby, it's not very easy. I used to sweep up the baby and take him for a walk – and walk far enough away that she couldn't hear.

She did say sometime later, 'You did that on purpose, didn't you?' And I said, 'Yes, because you weren't giving the older one enough time. It wasn't your fault, you had this screaming baby.'

grandmother of two

Daughters and daughters-in-law
Just as in pregnancy, giving advice is seen to be generally much easier with a daughter than a daughter-in-law:

People who have sons all feel that they are at a remove, because they're the mother of the partner, and it feels more intrusive. You have to wait to be asked.

Daughters-in-law feel judged by their mothers-in-law. If the relationship is strong enough, it's all broken down in month four or five when the baby's screaming and the mother realises that any help is good help. But you have to go through that. Whereas, as a mother of a daughter, you pretty much can just walk in, but you've still got to be sort of egg-shelly with the partner.

grandmother of one

You've got to be particularly careful when it isn't your daughter. I don't want to fall out with my daughter-in-law. Her opinion is valuable and I have to make sure that that's appreciated.

I'm probably slightly more open with my son. I just say, 'What do you think – if you did this, would it be better?' I feel I can say it more easily to him than I can to her, although she's a really lovely girl. I don't want to be seen as interfering, I do understand that I have to take a back seat.

grandmother of one

This is a very sensitive area, where you tread very carefully! It's all about gauging what other people want and each family has been different. You're always on safer ground with a daughter. With our daughter, I always felt comfortable in giving advice, because she would ask for it. With the daughters-in-law, I think you're always slightly more uneasy.

grandmother of ten

There is a concern about the follow-on impact on the young people's relationship:

With a daughter, you can be more honest. With a daughter-in-law, you are worried about the relationship between her and your son, that it might cause strain between them. If you tell your daughter off, she wouldn't necessarily tell her husband about what you said, but a daughter-in-law would immediately go and tell her husband, 'Your mum did this' or 'Your mum did that!'

In our Muslim culture, a son-in-law has to be treated extremely well, because otherwise he's not going to treat your daughter well. So you have to be careful. I can't be bothered too much with that, but I do try to hold my tongue when my son-in-law's around.

grandmother of one

Changing views about managing children
Another problem is that many grandmothers realise that views about many aspects of child-rearing have changed since their time:

Things change. Like with the feed – we used to be able to make up the feed for the day, put them in the fridge. You can't do that any more because of the bacteria in the milk. When I had my first, it was lay him on his side, when I had my second it was lay them on the belly, put them at the bottom of the cot – it's all different. I did adapt, because maybe there's a reason for that.

grandmother of six

It's much more customary now for new babies not to sleep in their cots all day, but to be part of the family almost from the word go. You have to accept that things have changed. Just recently, they were popping their finger into the baby's mouth when she was crying and I didn't think that was hygienic. In my day, everything around a baby had to be absolutely sterile.

You don't know what they've been told at pre-natal classes or in their own reading about childcare. Maybe they've read that's an okay thing to do. You don't want to offend them.

grandmother of ten

The whole idea of safety has so totally changed. You can't just put your child in a chair that you hook on to the back of your car and go off somewhere – it's got to pass all sorts of safety restrictions. It would be considered strange to let your child out all day and not know what he was doing. All sorts of things, the whole thinking has changed.

grandmother of eight

While many grandmothers manage to adjust, others feel that they are considered very much behind the times:

Sometimes, when she's pulling her hair out, I'll say, 'I'm sorry, but I wouldn't do that. I'm going to tell you what I would do – and then I'll walk out and you can carry on doing what you're doing.' She'll say, 'It's not the same now.' You're instantly old-fashioned.

grandmother of two

Some comment on how the climate for child-rearing has changed:

When my children were young, and indeed when I was young, there wasn't the emphasis on youth that there is now. Children were, quite often, 'seen and not heard', as they say. There was no adolescence as such – there was a transition from youth almost immediately to adulthood with responsibility and duty. Children were necessary and loved, but not made a great deal of.

Now, of course, we've almost gone too far in the sense that everything turns on children – perhaps we've gone a bit too far down that road.

grandmother of ten

Parenting is very different now. I think it's gone too far. Children now have too much choice. I can remember getting very cross with my son when he was young, shouting at him and insisting that he do what I said. Whereas the way that would be parented now is very different. They would not have nearly as much choice as children would have now. We would be the bosses and tell them what to do.

grandmother of two

Looking after the grandchildren
The question arises of how the grandmothers deal with their grandchildren when they are looking after them – in their children's ways or their own. Most say they try to fit in with what their children would like:

I clearly support everything her mother wants when my teenage granddaughter is rebellious, but she wouldn't really expect me to police it in the same way that her mother does. But if she said she's not allowed to do this, that, or the other, then of course I would honour all those rules.

grandmother of one

When they were small, I tried to keep as close to what they were used to as possible, so they didn't have many different regimes. They were being looked after by the other grandparents as well, so if we were all managing in totally different ways, they'd have three to contend with. And if you've got two parents, you've got two further ways of doing things anyway – I don't think you want six different ways of doing things.

grandmother of two

Some grandmothers sound as if they are almost frightened of going against the parents:

Being a grandmother, you don't have to make the decisions for them. If it's a serious decision, it's their mother who has to do that, not me. I can stand in the background and put my piece in and get shot down or not. They can come to me and say, 'Mummy said this' or 'Mummy said that'. I do try and back her up, because it's more than my life's worth not to! She's very sensible, so whatever she says is usually right.

grandmother of two

Because of the parents' strict views on sweets and biscuits, I wouldn't dare give the grandchildren any at all. But I've got a local shop where they make extremely delicious chocolate cupcakes and that's been allowed, as of about a year ago, but only for the oldest one. If we make cake for a birthday, we can have chocolate cake with good icing on top.

grandmother of three

Some say they do things their way as a matter of course:

I look after them my way, how I did mine. I said to their mums, 'If you don't like it, then I can't be looking after them – I have to do it my way.' But obviously, I will do certain things if they want me to do it for them.

grandmother of six

And some would check, if in doubt, with the parents:

It's a normal part of your interactions with small children that you say why this is a good thing or that's a bad thing. Why you should be nice to your sister or why you should forgive her for something. The parents do that as well. We're all involved in the same enterprise. I'm quite careful to say, 'You need to ask Mummy and Daddy about that' or 'Well, I don't think your Mum would like that and she's already told you off…'

grandmother of two

One grandmother notes that she will break the rules in a good cause:

Their mother has a rule that you never eat in front of TV and, at their home, it's in a separate

TV room. In my house, I follow the same rule, but if there's some very good programme on and my grandson wants to watch it, I'll take the food and I'll put it on his lap. So he knows that we are not rigid.

grandmother of two

Spoiling

Grandmothers are generally famous for spoiling their grandchildren and they don't disagree:

I probably let them get away with more than their parents do. It's so much easier – and you regard it as part of the grandparent's privilege that you are allowed to spoil them a little bit. You might let them have sweets more often than their parents would. Or you might let them get away with something.

It's only trivial things, really. Because it matters so much when it comes to morality and behaviour that the parents are getting it right – you have to support them.

grandmother of two

Aren't nannies allowed to spoil their grandchildren? I think so – a little bit. You tend to give in to them a little more than perhaps you do to your own children. Because you've not got the responsibility of bringing them up. So, where daddy might say no to her for biscuits, I might give her one. If she gets told off, she'll just run to me for a cuddle and I just cuddle her, whether it be right or wrong.

grandmother of one

Some suggest that spoiling is not really the right concept:

I don't like the word 'spoil'. I don't want to 'spoil' them. I'm aware that I could give them too many material things and I don't think that would help. I could spoil them by giving them too much time – that would be all right, that wouldn't be spoiling. It's not 'spoil' – you 'shower them with love'.

grandmother of two

How can you spoil your grandchildren? That's not spoiling them, that's loving them – and that's what grandparents are for. But they know they can't step over the line, I have my rules. They are certain things, like washing their hands when they go to the toilet. But, basically, I'm one of those nans who like to play.

grandmother of two

I certainly have been accused of spoiling – I'm sure my daughter has said it when her daughter was a lot younger, but I'm not sure it was totally true. If she would be difficult when she went home, it would be because I'd 'spoiled' her. But, in reality, when a child goes home, there's always a little settling-in period.

grandmother of one

Involvement in discipline
Some grandmothers instinctively avoid getting involved in disciplining their grandchildren:

As a grandmother, I would never, ever tell my little granddaughter off or smack her – I just don't think it's my place to do it. If she was touching pans or light sockets, I'd stop her and tell her it was dangerous, but for telling her off, I'd let her mum do that. You see some grandmothers that scream at their grandkids and you think, 'Oh, that poor kid.'

grandmother of one

I don't punish her. My daughter would set the boundaries and if I was babysitting at her house, I'd say 'No, you know you're not allowed to do that'. She wasn't allowed to be totally cheeky or destructive.

grandmother of one

Some seem happy to tell their grandchildren off, but nothing more:

If I think they're doing something wrong, I'll tell them. And my kids are quite happy with that. They've even said that I should smack them, if I think they needed it, but I've never had to. And I don't get the nasty bits, they don't really fight or argue a lot round me. They might be scared of me, because I've got quite a deep voice. If I've said, 'Don't do it', they don't.

grandmother of six

I'm not afraid to speak my mind. I think the closer you are to your grandchildren, the more you can speak to them. If you talk to some, they'll take it as an offence, or their parents will. Like, why are *you* telling them that? That's my job. But the closer you are, they're like your own children, you can speak to them – there's more freedom.

grandmother of seven

The grandchildren respect me, because if they're naughty, I'll just look at them, and that's enough – 'She's looking at us. Better behave yourself!' Just a look. They know where I'm coming from.

My upbringing in Barbados was much different from here. They could smack you at home, but they can't smack you over here, because the government says you can't smack kids, we'll put you in prison and all that. Over there, even the teachers used to smack us. And your parents would agree to it.

grandmother of ten

Some grandmothers set their own rules from time to time:

Just once, when she was about 14, I refused to take one grandchild out until she changed her clothes. What she was wearing seemed very inappropriate. I said, 'It looks like you've got your tights on, you haven't got a skirt on.' She said she didn't have a skirt she could wear, I said I wouldn't take her out then, looking like that. There were a lot of tears and shouting, but she did go up and get changed and we did go out. She's always a little bit of a rebel.

grandmother of eleven

Discipline gets complicated where families have differing views but spend a lot of time together:

My two-year old grandson gets away with a lot more with me than he does with his mum, because I just give in to him all the time, whereas

129

his mum doesn't. He's very boisterous and does naughty things, like chucking toys at my telly, and he gets told to stop, stop, stop. In the end, she'll put him on the naughty step, perhaps three times a week.

I have to keep out of the way, because he'll tell me he'll be good now and I want to get him off. He plays us off against each other. She says she can't give in, because when they go home, she's the one who's got to deal with him.

grandmother of one

My grandson is more relaxed with me and he never cries. I don't scold him much. He doesn't need it. He's a lovely little boy and he does listen. And when he's naughty, it's not serious naughtiness – he's making lots of noise and if you ask him to be quiet, he will give one loud bang, but he will stop.

I notice his mum and dad do tell him off. For example, his mum will say it's bedtime, but he wants to play outside. I'll let him stay that extra five minutes and say, 'Let him have a little more time. He likes to be outside.' But she'll say, 'No! Come in right now. You've got to listen to me!' They get a little bit of leeway from a grandmother.

grandmother of one

The occasional grandmother, however, is not so reluctant:

They've both felt the back of my hand, which I know you're not supposed to do these days.

Only once, but they have now understood that if you make Granny really cross, she will slap you. Normally I do it with words.

I was talking with my son recently about parenting and he said they were really scared of me when they were little, but they knew where the lines were. I had to work and couldn't afford to have them running rings round me. I never belted them in cold blood or anything like that.

grandmother of two

Parents don't care for their children or grandchildren in this country. Caring is not buying them £100 shoes, it's making sure that they eat the right food, they do the chores, do what they are supposed to do. And if they do wrong, tell them off, but with love – not screaming and shouting at them.

You need to explain why you are telling them off and then they will learn. It's spoiling children to let them keep on doing naughty things. A smack will stop them from doing a worse thing tomorrow.

grandmother of three

Helping with problems
On the other side of the coin, grandmothers are often able to help their grandchildren with problems. They recount examples of how they have helped in different ways.

Issues or problems at home

Where there are problems at home, grandmothers are an obvious source of help:

> The children will say 'Daddy got angry'. The younger one tends to say it more spontaneously. The older one knows that there are certain things you don't say, you don't need to tell Grandma, you don't need to upset anybody. But it just comes out. It's usually the same type of thing, the parents' arguments. They are upset and I tell them that they can come and talk to us anytime.
>
> ### grandmother of two

> I've had my grandchildren come and say, 'My dad and mum won't let me do this'. I'll sit them down and ask them what happened – what did their mum say? what did their dad say? And if they said they couldn't have something they wanted, like an iPad, I'd say, 'Well, perhaps they haven't got the money to get it. And maybe if you behave yourself a bit more and do what they ask you, instead of just taking things for granted, maybe you'll get that thing.'
>
> ### grandmother of seven

Or they are keen to be willing to be seen in this light:

> I'm just part of their life – somebody they know loves them whatever they do. I'm not going to be shocked by anything. They know that whatever they tell me, it wouldn't make any difference to me. I would help them. If it was something terrible – if they committed murder, I would help them. I would be horrified at what they'd done,

but I would still try and help and I would still love them because it is unconditional. That is what love is about, isn't it?

grandmother of two

Understanding themselves
Grandchildren of different ages may have a range of concerns and anxieties, where grandmothers can help:

Teenage children may not want to say things to their mum, which they may say to the grandparent. They tell me things, small things, like my granddaughter told me about how she's very upset over a friend at school, because she said something that made her unhappy. I asked her why she said it, maybe she had a reason. And then we talked and it came out who did what.

Later, I told my daughter and she hadn't known. Mothers are so busy in their lives, like we were busy with our lives, whereas we now have the time. My daughter didn't get cross, but said she would try to find a way of raising the issue.

grandmother of two

My 14-year-old granddaughter and I do talk. She quite often mentions that she's thinking about when she leaves home and what she wants to want to do. She asks me what I did when I left home, what I wanted to do and so on. That's quite nice, that she's interested in me as a whole person, not saying I'm old and unable to tell her anything. She'll tell me a bit about her friends, but she doesn't want to tell me about boys or anything.

grandmother of three

One entry into their world was a very significant conversation I had with my grandson when he was four. He was going through a stage of worrying that his mother would die – he asked me about death, he wanted to know what happens when we die. I said, 'Some people believe we carry on and have a different sort of life after we're dead, and some people think that we don't – that we just die and then there's nothing. And some people think there's heaven.'

He was actually worrying not just about death, but about separation from his mother. He said, 'If Mummy dies, I want to die at the same time' and I tried to explain to him very gently that, as he got older, Mummy wouldn't be the only force in his life, that he might have someone else he was very close to.

grandmother of two

I do tell them what I think about their choice of boyfriends. If somebody's not right, I will say they deserve better. I always say to them, 'Don't love a man more than you love yourself. Let them love you more and you won't get hurt so much.' I tell all women, fall in love, it's great, but please don't love them more than they love you.

grandmother of two

Sometimes, such concerns are of a practical nature:

Last week, I had my granddaughter with me and I told her all about periods. I explained to her what it was and all that. We were doing a biology lesson. Her mum may have told her, but I just asked her to remind me to discuss it with her mum, because they are due to go on a long trip 'We must tell Mum to carry some spare pads in case you start your period when you're away.' We can talk.

grandmother of two

Sometimes, grandchildren can reveal something even if they do not say it outright:

Once, my little granddaughter wanted to play schools and she was giving me a red circle, equivalent to a red football card. Every time I opened my mouth, it was wrong and I got a red circle and then I had to go to the headmistress and be told off for bad behaviour – and I hadn't done anything.

I thought about this afterwards and what it says about her experience at school. She loves school, but I think I was getting the shadow side of school – you have to do what you're told a lot and you might not like that too much. Because I was playing a new girl, I said I wouldn't come back to school tomorrow, I didn't like it here, and she said I could have a sweet if I would.

grandmother of two

Confidences are less common where there is infrequent contact:

They don't confide in me very much. I see them for short periods and I'm usually seeing them all together. One older one has been down here on her own and we've been out for a day to do something together. I might find a little bit out about how she's living her life and what her boyfriend is, but on the whole, they don't confide in me.

I think it's partly because they're able to talk within the family, they don't need to talk so much to me.

grandmother of eight

Wider questions

Of course, not all questions concern deep problems. Some grandchildren simply like to ask their grandmothers about the world around them:

One of them come home from school, and she said, 'Nan, were you in the war? Can you tell me any stories about what happened?' Which I did. I was telling her about when we were in the shelters. And I told her about being on rations and we were only allowed about four ounces of butter a week and things like that. She wrote it all down, put it all into a story and she got a prize in school for it.

grandmother of seven

The older one went through a 'why' phase. 'Why are you driving home this way?' 'Because the road down there is going to be very busy today and I don't want to get stuck in the .jam.' 'Why?' 'I don't really like sitting in traffic jams.' 'Why?' 'I can think of better things to do?' 'Why? 'Have a peppermint. Shut-up!'

grandmother of two

Chapter 6
The Image and Role of Grandmothers

Grandmothers have a number of possible roles in their grandchildren's lives. This chapter starts with the image of grandmothers and then explores how they actually see their role.

The image of grandmothers

The traditional image of a grandmother is a little old lady with nothing much to do with her life, aside from knitting or stroking the cat. Some put this clearly into words:

> There's the classic image that they're a little bit sweet, a little bit grey, a little bit doddery, a bit fatter – they're slower, they're wiser, they're kindly. Probably less active, probably less worried.
>
> *grandmother of two*

> My first reaction when I heard I was going to be a grandmother was, oh God, that's not very sexy. I was in my fifties and I was having a relationship with someone whose comment was, 'I've never been to bed with a grandmother.' I just told him he could have a new experience – and if he fancied going to bed with me one day, just because my daughter's given birth overnight, why not the next?
>
> I'm no longer with him, but his daughter's delivered two children since then, so he has become a grandfather.
>
> *grandmother of two*

One grandmother feels this general image devalues grandmothers and, in any case, is not based on reality:

I don't think grandmothers are valued enough. They tend to be seen as a little old lady with grey hair – that's totally out of touch with how people are. They say 70 is the new 50. You've got old people doing lots of things, we're working older as well, so it's not really caught up with how things really are.

I get very annoyed when I'm listening to the radio – a commentator said to some woman, whose husband had left and she had child care problems, why doesn't your mother do it? Well actually, most grandparents are working themselves and paying a mortgage themselves.
grandmother of three

One woman describes how she tried to fit herself into what she felt to be the classic image:

I was 50 and kind of astonished to find myself being a grandmother. One doesn't see oneself in that role, really. I went out and bought myself a suit and when I got home, I realised in the back of my mind that it was a suit that grandmothers would wear. I was never able to wear it. It was a kind of heather-coloured tweed. And it immediately 'grandmothered' me.

Then I thought, no, no, I don't have to do this! I hung on to the suit for quite a time, because it was quite nice, but every time I put it on, it felt completely wrong – I didn't feel I was that person. Of course, I hadn't changed, I was still the person I was, so there was no need to change the way I thought about clothes. I expect it went to Oxfam eventually and some other grandmother picked it up.

grandmother of eight

An unconventional woman describes how her young granddaughter saw her:

When she was about seven, they had to write about their grandmother at school. She starts of by saying, 'My Grandma is not your average grandma. She's got modern hair, she wears make-up, she paints her toenails and she always looks as though she's going to smile.' At the bottom, she put, 'And my grandmother has a special place in my heart that nobody else could ever fill.'

grandmother of two

A key part of the image of grandmothers is that they are old, however that is defined. But not only do many older women not *feel* old, many are indeed not that old at all. For these, telling other people that they are a grandmother brings a pleasurable response:

The word 'grandmother' seems so ageing. When I was first a grandmother, my daughter was twenty, I was in my thirties. I always thought it was quite funny. When I said, 'This is my granddaughter', absolutely everybody would say, 'You're not old enough'. It was fantastic. And you have much more energy to enjoy them, a lot more stamina. The drawback is that you still have to make money and worry about the roof and everything.

grandmother of one

People say to me, 'You don't look old enough to have a granddaughter'. It makes me feel nice that they think I'm still young – a lot of people put a perception on grandmothers as being quite old. In my mum's day, it was unheard of to be pregnant at a young age and have a young grandmother. Now, it's changed, I know one who's 38.

grandmother of one

When I tell people that I've got grandsons of that age, they say, oh no, you can't – you don't look old enough. I love it. It was one of the best things about being a mum at 21, because it's actually flattering for me. I've got a 34-year-old child, and people always say that can't possibly be. So that's nice.

grandmother of three

Own grandmothers

One source of the image of a grandmother is a woman's own grandmother. Some have strong memories and feel that they have been influenced by the nature of their own grandmother. Food is clearly part of many memories:

My grandmother was a typical head of the family. She was the woman everyone worshipped – the main character, the matriarch, the power. She was quite severe, but there was also a softness and tenderness about her. She became my role model in many ways. Her role was to keep everything in order in her house and cook delicious food.

She always had something special for me when I went there. I try to give that to my grandson. She used to boil milk so the cream settled, then gather that layer by layer in a plate, and put honey on it with nice bread. It was the most delicious thing in the world. An act of complete love.

grandmother of one

We used to love it if we had to stay the night at our grandparents. The omelettes for breakfast – I can still taste them! They had a vegetable patch and my grandfather used to take us out and invite us to choose a carrot and we'd just pull it out of the ground and wash it and it was all crunchy. My grandmother was very grandmotherly, hands on. I try to do things like that when I visit – I always go with a tin of homemade biscuits, because my grandmother always used to come over with stuff like that.

grandmother of five

My granny was a lovely woman back in Barbados. One day, she wasn't well, and none of her own kids were at home. I passed by and made her a cup of tea and gave her something to eat – and for that, she give me a baby chicken. I took it home to Mum and called it Peggy. We had to raise it – and when it got bigger, we ate it one Sunday for dinner. The way I am, it came from my Mum and my Gran.

grandmother of ten

But there are also other qualities:

> My father's mother died when I was about 9. I loved her to bits. She was a complete Cockney – she always had loads of beads and you could hear the beads rustling together. She was a really great character. It was always fun when she came round. I can remember my mum and her really laughing when they were shelling peas or things like that.
>
> And she used to tell my dad off, which was even better – she actually hit him once, a clip round the ears! Perhaps I get my sense of fun from her.
>
> *grandmother of three*

> We had a lot of contact with my mother's mother. She was quite grand – tall, big-boned, always dressed very smartly and dignified. Family was very important to her. She was very keen that we should only go out with anybody that she approved of. Anytime we had a boyfriend, she would say, 'Do we know his family?'. You always knew that she had a deep affection – taking a great interest, expecting the best of behaviour from us – but she wasn't cuddly. Quite a lot of my feelings about being a grandparent probably come from her.
>
> *grandmother of ten*

> They were very different, but very instrumental in my life. I was close with both of them. One was maternal, softer, housewifely, the other one was a Victorian lady. With her, I knew that I'd better sit up straight and behave myself, but I knew she loved me.

I do sometimes think I'm a bit like the Victorian one. I say to the grandchildren, 'Don't walk around my room eating your tea – sit at the table.' You learn that respect and knowing when you can do things. When they go out into the big, wide world, they've got to live with all the different people and they've got to respect them.

grandmother of two

The occasional woman feels she learned how *not* to be a grandmother:

I didn't really like my grandmother. She was a hard woman, very abrupt. I used to have to go every Saturday to the butcher's for her, and if it was cold out, she would stick one of these really hot peppermints in my mouth before I went, which I spat out outside. She wasn't cuddly and my mum wasn't either – maybe that's rubbed off on me a bit, because I'm not naturally affectionate, I wasn't very cuddly.

I try to be different with the grandchildren. I cuddle them and kiss them and tell them I love them. I didn't get that.

grandmother of eight

But some never knew their grandmothers for one reason or another. They tend to feel some loss:

I only knew one of my grandmothers. She was very elderly and she had been very dominant in my father's life. She hated my mother because she was married to her son – it was one of those.

So that was the only personal experience I had of grandmothers.

grandmother of two

My father's parents had died, my mother's mother was still alive, but she was pouring tea into the sugar bowl, I think she had Alzheimer's, so she wasn't there for me to relate to. Her body was there, but not much else of her mind was alive.

grandmother of two

And in some families, the loss is felt very deeply:

My father's whole family were killed in the Holocaust, the parents and the siblings, so we've got this missing bit. It was never talked about. My father's distress dominated our home and was very oppressive. I know lots of people were killed, but it's still difficult for *me*.

In our household, there was a lot of stifling anxiety, creating an unbearable tension. When I was a child, I felt I needed to get out, but I didn't know how. It's always been a struggle for me, this claustrophobia, feeling blocked in.

grandmother of three

Own mothers as grandmothers and mothers
Of course, by the time a woman is a grandmother, she has also normally seen her own mother in this role. Some talk about the importance to them of her example:

When I had my children, my mum lived across the road and she came over to me a lot. She'd come and see the baby, take her out, buy her things. If I needed her, my mum was there. If we were short of a bit of money, she would lend us some. It was nice to know that you had a grandmother that you could fall back on for help and support and just be there.

grandmother of one

My mother was definitely a grandmother to my children. She was great. She lived round the corner, so she was very close by and she was very involved. I wasn't living with the father of my children and I was working, so they used to go and visit her a lot. And they could take their friends there. Even if we weren't getting on particularly well, it was a practical thing.

grandmother of three

Some want to pass on to their grandchildren the mothering that they got from their mothers:

My mum was a really good, loving mum. When I speak to friends, they never had the love that I had. And I always thought if I ever had kids, I would really wrap them in love. She did it all on her own with three children. Her mum and dad disowned her, because of my dad being black, and she went through a lot of stigma. Everyone knew how much she loved us.

grandmother of six

And some consciously try to be different:

My mum was never physically affectionate. I don't think she ever gave me a hug and she certainly never told me she loved me, ever. She was very Victorian in that way. I made up my mind very young that when I had children I would be completely different. I made a very conscious decision to be very affectionate, and cuddly, and tell them that I loved them. And I still am.

grandmother of three

If anyone told my mum that I'd done something wrong, she wouldn't wait to hear my side. Straightaway there's lashes, using anything she could put her hand on. Much later, I told her I would never bring up my kids like that, because I would always wait to hear their side first. And that is what I've done – I hear their side of the story first before I beat them.

grandmother of ten

My mother was very cold. I put her on a pedestal, because she was very pretty and I was so proud to show her to my friends. It's only when I had my own daughter that I realised that I never had this *love* that pours out of you. I don't ever remember my mother telling me I was pretty, she never said about anything I did, 'That's great!'.

She was not a good grandmother. When I presented my little baby to her the first time, she looked at it and went 'Mmm', like here's a bloody nuisance. Her mentality was that it was going to interrupt my career.

And she never looked at my daughter with love. She was always criticising her. She lived far enough away, so she didn't have to see her much and she didn't want to. I used to invite her to come and she would suggest a date two weeks ahead and would sigh. Like she's doing me a big favour coming to London. She thought you mustn't have fun.

grandmother of two

Kinds of grandmother

Grandmothers could be categorised around a range of different features, but probably the most common is how involved they are with the grandchildren. Often, this is raised in terms of the amount of childcare they provide.

Providing childcare or not

Clearly, some grandmothers see their role as providing childcare on a regular basis, either full or part-time:

Being a granny did influence my decision to retire, because there weren't enough days in the week. I was there when needed, I hope. Certainly, not once a week or anything fierce like that. But when the second came along, she needed to go back to work four days a week. They could only afford two days of nursery, so his mother does Tuesdays and I do Wednesdays.

grandmother of two

I was hands-on. My daughter was making a career for herself in business with her husband, so I had my grandchildren more or less all the time. I was the one who would rush out to pick them up from school. And every single weekend, the two of them used to come and stay with me.

They used to fight to come on their own. They each wanted to have me for themselves, to talk to and whatever. If one was going to a party with school friends, the other would say, 'Oh, I'll go to Grandma's on my own, then.' I could concentrate more on one, of course. You can concentrate more on the bedtime story with one, not trying to dodge between two bedrooms.

grandmother of two

Others are quite the opposite, establishing from the start that they will not be sucked into a babysitting role:

I never did regular childcare. I didn't want to be a child-minder. Only once, for one of the girls who was in a nursery and I could give one day a week. But I have never gone in for 'looking after'. I do not go out for three days a week to anybody's house. I had my own career and I felt that that wasn't what I wanted to do. School holidays, yes. But on a regular basis, no.

grandmother of ten

I made it quite clear from the start, I'm not the unpaid babysitting help. I don't really like babies, I want to see my grandchildren, but I want to *want* to see them. I don't want to have them foisted on me so that I'm so knackered, I want to throw them out the window. I try to avoid a whole day with both of them together, as they niggle each other and fight when they are tired.

I talked it through with my family – there's no hidden agenda like 'Oh, Mum says she'll babysit, but she's never available when we ask.'

We've worked it out between us. I don't dislike being a grandmother – and I didn't *want* to dislike being a grandmother.

grandmother of two

When the first one was born, I said, 'I'm not a babysitting grandmother.' Which meant that I didn't want to permanently regularly say that every Thursday I could be a babysitting grandmother. I couldn't, because I was still earning a living. Of course, I did look after them at times or in the evening.

grandmother of eight

Even one afternoon a week is quite a commitment. Once you do that, you have to honour it, even if you're not well or you want a holiday. I have friends who feel they're being asked to do too much – it's a real bind and it exhausts them. I've had none of that, there have been no excessive demands placed.

grandmother of two

This raises the question of whether grandmothers provide this service because they feel they *have* to or because they *want* to. Some are clearly in the latter camp:

I do it because I want to. My husband comes with me sometimes. It's lovely, we both enjoy it. Yesterday, I was looking after two of them, we were collecting another one from school, and I took the baby out to give my daughter a rest. He was quiet and slept and the older two were very thrilled to have their new cousin, they were showing all their friends.

grandmother of eleven

People say, 'Don't you get fed up?', but I don't –
I love it. If they want me, I'm there. I don't feel
used. When my daughter asks me to have the
children, she always asks if it's all right with me
– and if it wasn't, I would say no. Afterwards,
she will bring me a box of chocolates, and thank
me. I don't work anymore, so I can give more
time.

grandmother of eight

I help my daughter a lot because I *want* to be
involved, not that she's telling me to do things. I
don't feel put-upon. My husband tells me
sometimes, 'You are being taken for granted,'
but he's wrong. I can say 'no' if I want, but I
don't want to, because I enjoy doing it. So, what
is the problem?

grandmother of two

But there are others who feel put-upon by the
demands placed on them:

I had him here all the time leading up to
Christmas. And, as much as I love them both to
bits, come Boxing Day, and they were going
home, I felt whew, I can get my house in order.
I'd let them have a good time, toys everywhere.
It's very quiet after they've gone. But I need to
have them out, just to get my head back together
again. I could say no. There has been the odd
night where she's wanted to go somewhere, and I
have told her no.

grandmother of one

When my great-granddaughter got christened, for the whole week leading up to her christening, they were here. I did all the baking for them. Then we all went on to the christening and people were asking about the cakes and wanting me to make one for them. They were all proud of me – 'This is my nan, the best nan in the world!'

I felt proud at the time. But since then, I haven't seen them. I think they used me. If there's another one, I won't be doing all this baking. You can use me once, but not twice.

grandmother of ten

I felt like a babysitter – not a grandmother. I would have liked to be a part of them coming home from work, having dinner – them doing it and me being the grandmother. I would've been there at weekends, going out every now and then with them. Instead, when I'm finished there, I can't wait to go home, because I feel like I've done a *job*. I don't want to feel like that. I want to lie on the floor and play with them.

grandmother of two

And some are clearly highly ambivalent:

If I look after the baby, they should be very grateful. It should be their pleasure, not mine. In fact, we all know that's not true – it is *my* pleasure – but my pleasure has got a limit. I can't physically give more than what I'm giving now.

I printed out my own weekly programme, explaining when I was free and that they had to collect the baby at one o'clock at the latest. I can't look after him for the whole day, although they were hoping that I could. And I need one full day to myself. I've set my own boundaries.

grandmother of one

One grandmother who lives very far away from her grandchildren muses on the advantages:

The advantage of not having our children around is we never get put-upon. I never feel used. When we get together, they're really pleased to see us. It's short and intensive and it's planned. We know when we're going to see them.

I wouldn't like to be the kind of grandmother where I had to see them every day – we like having our own life. I go out and see friends, we go away a lot. If they were all living nearby, I'd feel I'd have to be quite organised, picking the kids up from school. I wouldn't like to be on call all the time. It's a bit selfish, but if you don't have your own space then you get a bit suffocated.

grandmother of five

The many aims of grandmothers

But there is more to being a grandmother than providing – or not providing – childcare. Some give a lot of thought to the question of what they are there to do.

Supporting the parents

Very commonly, grandmothers see their principal role as providing support to their son or daughter in their parental role. This may be a matter of practical help:

I try to be supportive both of the grandchildren and their parents. It's more for the parents, because they make the requests. If they phone and say 'I have a problem, can you help?', I do my very best to help. I feel pleased that she feels able to ask. And if ever I can't do something, I say so.

grandmother of eleven

I try to catch moments when I ought to be there. I try to gauge her tone of voice, as much as anything. If I offer something and she says 'No, no, it's absolutely fine', there are several ways of saying that. It can be that it *is* absolutely fine, so just bugger off. Or there's the 'Well, it ought to be all right, but I am tired and yes, it would help if you did do so-and-so, but I don't want to ask you.' Unspoken.

And then there's the 'No, it's absolutely fine. *Of course*, we can manage.' At which point, I get in the car saying, 'I don't care if you can manage, I'll come over in any case.'

grandmother of two

Or it may be a matter of providing some reassurance:

One of the big things about being a grandmother, is telling the parents they're getting it right, reassuring them. Sometimes my daughter will say she feels she is doing it all wrong and I will remind her that she can't do everything and is doing things a lot better than I would've done. They worry a lot and you have to say, 'It doesn't matter. I worried about that, but it will sort itself

153

out.' I think all of that reassurance is really, really helpful.

grandmother of two

Helping the grandchildren

But some grandmothers think much more closely in terms of the role they play with the grandchildren themselves at different stages in their lives.

Some have a strong wish to be involved in developing the children's minds:

Learning is the important thing for me. I have planned with my daughter to give him the best education, as much as we can afford. I believe in the old style of academia, that they are ready to learn everything from a very early age – maths, sports, languages, art and music. So, my role is teaching and kind of play.

But in order to do that, we have to practise, putting time and discipline in. My daughter and I decided that we would start doing it early. We take the baby and the pushchair and, every now and then, go to visit different museums. Just to become accustomed going into places with the baby.

grandmother of one

I like to help them grow. I find it very exciting, the way my grandson's mind works. He's a very able child. It's wider than just intellect, it's this curiosity – he thinks very fast, at a level that's way above his age.

And it's the way he connects things up, he's very wise. He's my flesh and blood – I suppose it echoes in me. I've loved ideas and he loves ideas. I watch his mind expanding and his interest in everything around him. His wanting to know, his wanting to understand and his amazing ability to understand.

grandmother of two

One notes, however, that one can take this concern too far:

We're always busy doing things. I feel I have to teach them things, educate them as much as I can, like going to visit galleries and museums. Sometimes when they come, I fill the time with things to do, and then when they leave, I think maybe I didn't sit down enough and feel their energy and just be with them calmly. They are very sensitive children and I think I should allow these moments – not miss them.

grandmother of two

A concern with the minds of the grandchildren may also extend to their spiritual needs, albeit with very different perspectives:

I guided my grandson on right and wrong in life. We read the Bible a lot. I got him involved in the Church and he went to a Roman Catholic primary school. I wanted him to fear God, because when you fear God you have wisdom. When you don't have it, you just behave any which way. I gave him a spiritual, moral background.

grandmother of three

I believe it's very important to pass on values. With the Muslim religion, you've got to do all the rituals. We pray five times. My little grandson has learned just by watching us. At home, when he sees us praying, he takes out his prayer mat and he does all the actions. And we have certain prayers that you read every night, that are in Arabic. He knows them and he's learning Arabic as well. That's very important, the religious bit.

In the Muslim faith, it's the women who teach the small children about religion and the fathers take over later on with the explanations and the history. I teach him a bit – not from the Quran as such, but our Prophet's name and what he did and little stories. He knows that Ramadan is coming up and that everyone's fasting and why. But he's a bit too young for very much.

grandmother of one

I would like to make sure they won't be indoctrinated into any faith. I find religious guilt very damaging. A non-believer is a freer individual. I don't want religious guilt to be planted into my grandchildren. They would become people led by the local priest to do what the he tells them. I want to help them to be themselves.

grandmother of five

In contrast, some see themselves as people who provide a sense of fun:

My son gave me a 'onesie' for Christmas – it is a cow costume, with a cow head and a cow tail and every so often I put it on and they will boss me around and I am the cow baby. They particularly like to be the mummy and the daddy – they will leave me to be babysat in the house on my own and go off. I'm told to go to sleep, or told to do this or that – something about role reversal. Instead of the adults telling you what to do, you tell the adult what to do.

grandmother of two

I'm purposefully trying to be fun. I learned to ride a motor bike a couple of years ago, and they thought that was great, and recently I got a wetsuit to go outdoor swimming with my daughter. So they think that's quite good fun.

grandmother of three

One describes stepping in when there are temporary difficulties:

The older one's nose was very out of joint at having a sibling for the first six months or so. The parents both told him – and tried to show him – that he was loved just as much as her, but of course it was difficult that someone had come and taken over Mummy. I was there once a week and I became 'his', it made him feel better to have his own person. After six months, there was a turnaround. He made it clear that he loved his baby sister.

grandmother of two

Fostering a sense of family

Many families are spread out geographically or simply too busy to come together very often. Another aim of grandmothers is to foster a sense of family, to ensure that different members of their family feel some sense of kinship with one another. Often, this seems to centre around food. In some cases, it seems to come easily:

Eating was a social thing, where we all sat down at the table when they were younger and talked – and I still feel that's very important. And no phones for the grandchildren. On the Friday night, or on the Sabbath, if they're at this house, they can't put their phones on – they're not allowed. One granddaughter told another, when she put her phone on at the table, 'We don't have uninvited guests at the table' – that's how we feel about it. I feel you should sit down and eat with your children and talk.

grandmother of eleven

Sometimes, it is more of a struggle:

We eat dinners at different times because they come in at different times and are all hungry. I said to them once that there should be a time, a family time, when we should all have a meal together. So, whenever we do weekends, we all sit as a family and we can talk. If we go there and my grandson is eating with his iPad and the earplugs in, I will say it is rude, he should be enjoying his food. And he puts it down.

grandmother of two

We make an effort sometimes to have a family lunch, which will involve my other children, so that they can have some bonding with the little grandchildren. They're all very friendly, but it's the only thing that keeps the family relationship going. If we didn't do it, we wouldn't see them much.

The parents always fuss about keeping a rigid routine. When they come here, they bring food for the children. I think they're concerned that ours might have too much salt or sugar. The children are very contented, very secure, but it does make it a bit difficult when they're stepping outside their routine.

grandmother of two

Long-term relationships

As grandchildren grow into their later teens and adulthood, grandmothers talk less about their purpose and more about how they simply enjoy their relationship with them:

I've got friends who say, 'I brought my own children up, I don't want to do childcare.' That's their personal choice, but they're missing out, because if you form a nice relationship with the grandchildren when they're young, that remains. The older grandchildren still phone up and chat. My husband is often in the town where my daughter is at university, on business, and my granddaughter comes to have lunch with him.

grandmother of eleven

I've never thought of myself as a 'grandmother grandmother'. I get on with all their friends. They'll phone me up and say, 'Grandma, we're going out for cocktails – come and join us.' Even quite late. I don't always go, sometimes I'll say 'I'm an old lady, I'm sitting here relaxing with the television – leave me alone' but they press me to get a taxi and come.

I sometimes join them at parties. Even years ago, they would come into the grown-up' room and say 'Grandma, come and join my friends, they all want to talk to you.'

grandmother of two

Some grandmothers of teenage children note that this is beginning to happen in their families, such as this Indian grandmother:

I wasn't even 50 when my grandson was born, so I've grown with them. My ideas are young and I've not been a strict grandmother, I've been more like a friend to them. So, they love coming here, they come all the time. My granddaughter comes every Friday night and stays over.

It's just so wonderful to have grandchildren around you. And to *do* things for them. Sometimes my granddaughter comes in late after swimming, and she's hungry. I always make her what she asks for – I'll say 'Okay, you go have a wash, put your nightie on, your puri will be ready.'

grandmother of two

And another:

We have always seen a lot of each other, sometimes every day. When my granddaughter was first born, I would go around to their house on my way home, to make sure that they'd eaten, because neither of the parents were working at the time. Later on, I had to change my lifestyle so that I could spend more time with them.

Now, I don't see them every day, but I've got keys to their house so I'll go feed the cat, do whatever – if they're there, it's a bonus. It's more likely to be my granddaughter there, and we'll have little chats.

grandmother of one

Some grandmothers like to think that their home will be a magnet one day, when their grandchildren are old enough:

She lives with her mother and her mother's husband, and she's sometimes annoyed about something or other. I've told her that when she's a bit older, she's welcome come and stay with me, even for a week. There's a spare room, 'You can just have some space if you want to.' She said she would think about it. That's my fantasy – that she would want to come and spend more time with me.

grandmother of three

I've worked out that I'm going to be the coolest granny in town, because I'm living bang in the city centre and they're living in a village. They'll come and crash at granny's – they don't have to get home. I think it'll be fun. I won't have to deal with their teenage angst – their mum will have to do that, so it'll just be nice. I'm here to do it.

grandmother of two

Some comment on the importance of giving the grandchildren time early on as a means of establishing a long term relationship, whether with teenagers or far beyond:

The thing you want from the beginning is that the relationship starts from when they are very little and builds up. You hear of a lot about children, maybe in their early teens, wanting to escape from the pressures of the parents, and they escape to granny, who will understand them, and so on. Unfortunately, I'll be pretty elderly by then, and couldn't give them very much.

grandmother of two

I collect rude poems, the sort of thing they learn in the playground. Things like 'Three fat ladies stuck in the lavatory, they were there from Monday to Saturday' – they're all lavatorial, there's nothing beyond that yet. She's only eight. I use that, which I used with my own children, so that they are free to talk to me about anything with me.

grandmother of five

Some feel this is just a matter of being known to them:

I never thought about it a great deal, but I wanted them to know me. I didn't want to be a distant person on the horizon, but to know me and for me to know them. That's the most significant thing.

grandmother of ten

Grandmothers are there to love them. To just be there, to tell them all the things that their mum and dad don't tell them. All the silly things in life. Like my granddaughter will ask silly questions like, 'Why does chewing gum stick to your shoes?' and her mum and dad tell her to be quiet, but I'll tell her 'Because people throw it on the floor.'

grandmother of two

Financial involvement
The 'bank of mum and dad' has become an increasingly familiar story and it often comes into play when grandchildren are born. The extent of the parental contribution varies with the nature of the respective circumstances. It may be simply a matter of buying occasional extras to help out young parents of limited means:

Being a grandmother is expensive. If we go out shopping and we see a toy, or some clothes, or even some baby milk or nappies, we pick it up for her. I didn't keep anything after I had my kids.

grandmother of one

Nearly every day I would do some kind of shopping. I was very happy being able to buy clothes – anything they needed.

grandmother of one

But it can also be helping with more sizeable expenses:

One grandson had hearing difficulties – he obviously was quite deaf – and we ended up paying for an operation. My daughter was going through all the National Health route, until I got exasperated because there was a long wait for an appointment.

I found a good paediatric ENT guy on the net and made a date for a diagnosis. She was very reluctant, but in the end, we paid – he couldn't start school when he was supposed to, he wasn't communicating enough. Now, he's a delight, he's talking away.

grandmother of two

Nowadays, education is the main thing. Colleges, universities – how they are going to manage it, it's very expensive. Whatever I have is going to go to them. I tell my daughter that I want her children to have a good education, to stand on their feet nicely. If times come hard, I just say, whatever I have is coming to you – use it for the children, it is for them.

grandmother of four

And some choose to help out financially where they feel it is appropriate:

I've never *had* to help them out financially. I've chosen to give money quite often, but nobody's asked me for it. If they've been here and seen something they wanted – 'Oh, Granny, you couldn't buy that for me, could you?' I've probably said yes. But nobody yet has been independent sufficiently long to require large sums from me.

We've tried to help the older grandchildren. For example, one granddaughter worked for six months to come over to England from Australia where she lives and we decided to give her a lump sum to top up all the hard work she'd done.

And we'd do that for everybody at an appropriate time, as long as it was agreed with the parents.

grandmother of ten

It can certainly add up:

We're involved quite a lot financially. I've never worked out how much, but it's a fair size I would guess. When my daughter stopped working, there was quite a big gap, so I pay for the boy's nursery fees and I give her a lump sum every month so she can get a few luxuries, face creams and that sort of thing. And I pay for their petrol when they make long journeys.

I just feel that the quicker they get on their feet, the better. Nobody ever gave us a penny – we just made do with what we could – but they have expectations, they don't adjust to the financial situation that they're in. They still carry on doing things as if they were earning two salaries.

grandmother of one

Chapter 7
The Impact on Other Relationships

When grandmothers think about their various relationships, their attention is principally focused on the grandchild or grandchildren. But in fact the presence of grandchildren affects many different relationships within the family. This chapter explores how these might change.

The son-in-law or daughter-in law (or partner)
Turn the word 'grandmother' around to a different vantage point and she becomes a mother-in-law. This has never had a good ring to it, but in fact the relationships of grandmothers to the partners or spouses of their children vary enormously.

The good stories
Some mothers-in-law get on very well with their son's or daughter's partner:

> One son's wife fits within our whole family very well – we've been very fortunate. We are welcome to pop in if we are visiting our daughter, because they live near each other. I have a nice relationship with her, which I think is to do with her, really. One of my friends has a very unpleasant daughter-in-law and for quite a few years she wasn't allowed to see the children. Now, she can, but they don't live very near, so it's only once or twice a year. It's very painful.
> *grandmother of eleven*

> I'm another mum to my daughter-in-law – she hasn't had her mum since she was 18 months old. Her mum walked out and left the four

166

children with the father. She was brought up by her nan and granddad in the house she's living in now. She is very affectionate and very giving to me.

grandmother of eight

My son-in-law and I are great mates. He's quite a character and great fun. He and my daughter were great friends before they got together and we were friends, too, back then. We're all very open – not your normal family. My daughter doesn't go in for dancing much and he'll say to me, 'Come on, let's you and I go and dance.' We have a great friendship.

We used to go on cruises, all five of us. The first night at the table, there would be other people there and when I came in all dressed to kill, my son-in-law would say, 'Oh, the old tart's here now!' The people at the table looked shocked, but they got used to us.

grandmother of two

One even refuses to use the term 'daughter-in-law':

I treat my daughter-in-law as a daughter. I told her parents 'I'm not her mother-in-law, I'm her mother-in-love.' I give her love, she is my daughter. I'm not an in-law. When they introduced me first time, they kept calling me 'mother-in-law' and I kept correcting them. I said, 'Please don't call me that.' So, they understood, and then they said, 'Her second Mum'.

grandmother of two

Some continue to get on with their child's partner or spouse even when the marriage (or relationship) has come to an end:

> My daughter's partner is really good with the baby. He gives my daughter money each month for whatever she needs. You can get some that don't – they just get a girl pregnant, then leave her to manage on her own. He has stuck by her. We still see him. He's said that we're really good and thanks us for what we do.
>
> ***grandmother of one***

> My son's partner is Dutch. They had a love affair and she got pregnant, but they weren't living together. She told me later that it wasn't an accident, she had wanted him to be the father of her child. And then they learned that it was twins. The relationship wasn't established and suddenly it was two! That relationship broke down quite early.

> I'd met her twice. That was fine, I've always got on very well with my two sons' girlfriends. And I could relate to her in so many ways, because I lived in Holland as a child but I hadn't been for *years*. So, it was like this huge surge of history for me, which was incredibly emotional for me. She reminded me of a younger me. I related to her a lot. It was quite extraordinary.
>
> ***grandmother of three***

Strained relationships
On the other hand, there are many very strained relationships:

She really values my grandmothering. She doesn't always value *me*, but she values me as a grandmother. I sometimes think she doesn't much like me as a person, which is probably about rivalry – mother-in-law, daughter-in-law stuff. Perhaps she felt that her husband was closer to me than to her when she was first with him. If I was someone else, she probably would like who I am.

I can feel quite shut-out at times. I'm welcomed as a baby-sitter, but they will go off on holidays with her parents, and we don't have anything equivalent. And there's loads of photos of the children around their house, some with the other grandparents, but there are none of us. When I realised it, I felt a bit pushed out.

I can remember arriving to be with the children and my daughter-in-law putting the baby down near me and looking at her face and saying, 'She's suspicious of you.' I thought, oh, thanks very much! It does help to say that.

grandmother of three

She went back to work and I went down there and babysat. When you're babysitting for a new born, you clean up. They were both working, I thought I'll cook their dinner, wash their clothes, I'd do little things and she would come home to a clean house. But it made her feel a bit uncomfortable and it became a competition: 'Does your mum think I'm dirty?' or 'Your mum's washing is better than mine.' It wasn't done like that.

She thinks I don't like her, but I'd give her a medal, gladly, for putting up with my son. I want to praise her and say, 'Oh, my God, no one would love him as much as you.'

grandmother of two

When the baby was eight months old, my husband and I treated them all to a holiday. The second night, I could hear them shouting. Shortly after, my son-in-law said to me, 'Your daughter's absolutely unbearable. Whatever I do is not good enough for her.' And I said, 'Do you realise that she's just had a baby? Maybe she needs a little bit more help?' He threatened to leave the next day, but he didn't, but he complained about everything – the table was wrong, the chair, the sun was too strong.

At the end of the fourth day, we had a real argument – he banged on the table and asked why did I have to offend people all the time. I said, 'I'm glad if have I offended you, because this might actually keep us even, after all the offences that you have given me and us during these eight months.'

grandmother of two

A frequent comment is that the spouse is very 'controlling':

My son's partner is a very controlling person. I don't want to be unfair, because she is very talented at her work and has been a very good mother. I know she is very fond of me, and I am of her, in many ways. The children are fine, but there is a controlling element which made it

uncomfortable for me to stay with them very
often.

grandmother of eight

His parents were far more involved than I was.
That was quite hard. It was to do with him –
controlling, aggressive, basically just wanted his
own family around. He had a very high-powered
job and just liked to be in charge of everything. I
think he very much looked down on me and my
husband, perhaps because my husband was
black, and he was a bit racist. It was *very*
difficult.

They're not together now and she's now got a
new partner, who's lovely. A nice guy, very
respectful to me.

grandmother of two

She's just a very controlling person about the
way she wants things to be, and so our
relationship with the children has been on their
terms, not ours. What has made it a bit sad is
that I'm aware that it can be different – my close
friend is endlessly looking after her
grandchildren.

What I miss, and what I would really like to have
had, and my husband too, would be to have our
own special, private relationship with the
children, which was *ours*. They're very friendly,
but our relationship is on the terms that the
parents have set up.

grandmother of three

Absent partners

Quite a frequent occurrence is an absent partner, particularly men. This means that there is no son-in-law (or daughter-in-law) with whom to relate. This is especially noticeable where a very young daughter has a baby:

> She was with him for three years, phoned him and told him at work that she was pregnant, and he never came back. It's hard to hear that. I look at my grandson every day and just think, 'Well, it's his loss.' He's had quite a few opportunities, he was sent texts about scan dates and to say that the baby had been born, and what hospital – and nothing. Until this day, he's never responded. It's hurtful.

> You know there's going to come a time where my grandson's going to start asking about his dad. I don't know what I'll tell him. I won't just say, 'Well, your dad didn't want to know.'

> He was the same age as my daughter, 22. We're looking out for him all the time, but we've never seen him. It's very sad. It's sad for my daughter to have been with someone for all those years and never thought for a minute that he was capable of doing something like that. I suppose he just didn't want to be a dad, he didn't want responsibilities, he didn't want to pay the child maintenance – there's probably a lot of reasons.
>
> > ***grandmother of one***

> I can't remember how old she was when they finally split. He only worked intermittently – he was one of these super play station players.

There came a time when she just couldn't stand it anymore. He was just not helping, because he was always staying up at nights playing play station, and sleeping during the day. That was pretty much during their entire relationship. He has now grown up and got a job.

grandmother of one

One Nigerian grandmother explains that neither of her daughter's partners lasted very long:

> The first one wanted a Nigerian marriage. In our tradition, if you want to marry, you have to go to the other family and introduce yourself, so they know who you are. The boy's mother didn't like the fact that my daughter was English. But my daughter was already pregnant. Nigerians used to think girls should be pregnant before they marry to show they are fertile.

> She was only 19 and said she wanted to kill herself. But she was the only thing I was living for. I just tightened my girdle and said, 'If you kill yourself, what do I do?' I brought her back to England, she had the baby and finished her A-levels.

> Then she met another Nigerian, and decided to marry him. She insisted he would never disappoint her. She went to America with him and became pregnant with twins. When she had them, she wanted to give them Ibo names, but he told her if she did that, it would be the end of the marriage. Perhaps for that reason, he divorced her. He left when the twins were three months old.

grandmother of three

Sometimes, however, there is an absent woman:

> I never liked my son's partner, the mother of one of my granddaughters. I never got on with her. She was a liar and not a very nice person. When my son broke up with her, to see my granddaughter I would've had to have dealings with her, so I was estranged from both for a long time. I didn't know where she was. It was hard.
>
> I was going to go to court to have access to her, but in the end I thought if I have access to her, I've got to have dealings with the mother – and I'd rather not have that. I thought, when she's old enough, she'll find me – and she did when she was about 20.

grandmother of eight

The son or daughter with the grandchildren

The presence of a grandchild means that there tends to be more contact not only with a son- or daughter-in-law, but also with the son or daughter. Some say that this has no effect on their relationship, because it was good in any case:

> We'd always been quite close because I'd brought them up practically on my own. I was divorced since the oldest was only seven and my daughter was only a year old. So, they only had me. My daughter's my rock. She does everything for me, nothing's too much trouble. They help me now, my kids.

grandmother of eight

My daughter and I always been very close. All through my last marriage, it was like there was just me and her, because my husband was off with other things most of the time. I'm in awe of her. If you've got a problem and ask her what to do, within a minute, she will get right to the centre of what is troubling you. All her friends go to her for advice. She's quite a special person. We have a lot of the same friends. Sometimes the generations stay all separate, but our family doesn't.

grandmother of two

Some say that the arrival of a grandchild has improved their relationship:

I think if they hadn't had children, they'd have wandered off into their own life, which would have become increasingly different. Not quite estranged – I'd have been there for them, they'd have been there for me, but we wouldn't have had to bump into each other so much. We shouldn't have had so much to do with each other, there wouldn't have been so much a big project for us to share.

Sharing it is a nice thing for her and it's something I'm keen to be involved with. But also, in our modern life, you can't actually raise children without the grandparent input anymore. Even with nannies and nurseries and everything, you have to have the back-up.

grandmother of two

It brought my son and me even closer. I thought it would be different, but my daughter-in-law needed me more. I'm really pleased. They went back to work and I had both their children until they went to school. They always stayed a couple of nights a week, they still do that now. They still come round.

grandmother of six

What has been positive about it all is I felt I lost my son between the ages of 17 and 27 in the sense that he wasn't terribly interested in coming home – he went to university, he was leading his own life, he was busy. He was perfectly happy, but you had to ring, you had to force yourself on him as a parent. I think sons often do that. But as soon as he had his own family, he did really want us. He wanted us to be part of his life again. So that's nice.

grandmother of two

Some comment that they feel their children appreciate them more:

Now my daughter is seeing how I look after her son. Grown-up children start thinking, we were like that – our Mummy has looked after us the way she's looking after *my* children now. And they start to realise what our parents have gone through to bring us up. I think they appreciate it more and more. We were always a close family, but they have more love for me now, seeing how they feel about their own children. That's our Mum now, she has done so much for us.

grandmother of four

My relationship with my daughter has become better. We are more on the same wavelength as two mothers, and she understands me better in regard to my behaviour towards her as a mother. Like making comments, giving instructions – she knows that I wanted the best for her, because she wants everything the best for her child. So, she can associate with that.

grandmother of one

But the occasional woman suggests that the existence of a grandchild has worsened the relationship:

My relationship with my son has become more distant since his second child was born. It feels sad. This could be that in order to be close to his wife, he has to be distant from me, because she seems to feel there's some rivalry between us, which I think creates rivalry between us. I think he found it very stressful doing his job and becoming a father. His wife had enormous expectations of sharing the children with him, she felt he wasn't doing enough.

I detected some bitterness towards me. I don't know whether that was, 'You didn't mother me like this' or 'I'm finding this role really difficult, trying to be a good father and my partner's expecting far too much of me and I can't do it.' If he hadn't had children, I think I would be closer to him. I'm valued as a grandmother, but I think the mother-son relationship has suffered.

grandmother of two

Although she was living with us, she was alone at home with the baby, because I went to work. She never forgave me for that. I said that I had a life of my own and that she must fit in with me a little bit. She thinks that we are selfish, that we

should all work around her and her children –
nobody gives them enough time. And then she
will say, 'Oh, I'm going out to dinner. Mum,
would you look after the kids?'

She thinks I'm to be the carer. I say, 'You're the
mother! You've got a young husband. You two
sort it out – don't involve me.' I've got a life of
my own and I've brought my children up. Now,
it's her turn.

grandmother of two

In one case, the situation seems to bring out earlier
resentments:

My son and his partner split up about a year after
the twins were born. He was having little times
with them on his own, but they're a handful and
it was all very fragile. I tried to remind him
about the children's needs, and he said, 'Don't
you tell me how to bring up children. You of all
people, how dare you tell me about bringing up
children!'

He has lots of resentment towards me to do with
my lifestyle when I was younger, not living with
his dad, and he was very aggressive about the
fact that I had other men in my life.

We've ended up having nothing to do with each
other. I was in a lot of pain about that. I can
communicate with his ex-partner and I've also
had contact with her mother. My main concern
was to keep the communication open with the
mother of his children. He severely resented that.
He thought that I shouldn't have anything to do

with her – and that I should, at all costs, support him. He'd say, 'Your first loyalty is to me, not to *my* children.' The whole thing was terrible, but I just thought that I had to do it.

grandmother of three

The other grandmother(s)

It is sometimes suggested that grandmothers can become somewhat competitive with the other grandmother, the mother of their son's or daughter's partner or spouse. They might compete for their grandchildren's affection or simply want to have equal time with them. There is the occasional admission of such feelings:

My son-in-law's parents hardly ever saw my beautiful grandchildren. They're both dead now, but they hardly ever saw them. Perhaps they spent more time with their daughter's children. They weren't bad grandparents, they loved them, but they didn't see them, they never took them out on their own, they never babysat them. That suited me. I didn't have to share with anybody. Lovely.

grandmother of two

If I had my way, I'd see my little granddaughter every week, but it doesn't happen like that. I might see her once a month. There's the other grandparents – you do not get a look in. Especially his mum. I won't say anything, because it's her son. And the grandfather's always with the child, walking her here, walking her there. Let them get on with it. When I see her, I'm happy. I don't interfere. I just take a backseat.

grandmother of ten

When my daughter finally had a boy, I felt a bit of competition with his mum. She never had any more children because she couldn't guarantee having a boy – that's her. I just felt, you never made that much a fuss over the little girl, but now the boy's come along, you show a lot more for him. In fact, he absolutely adores me, he tells me he loves me. I think it upsets her.

His sister once said to me, 'My Nana hates you.' It really hurt me, but I said, 'Does she? I really like her – give her a big kiss from me.' What else can you say? Just reverse it a bit. But then you realise, they aren't your kids, you have to step back. They're somebody else's, even though they're your child's kids, they belong to another family as well.

grandmother of two

But in contrast, there is also commonly a sense of working together to help the younger family. Sometimes, this concerns juggling child care:

The mum and dad of my daughter's partner were really, really good. Because the baby stays here and lives there, we have to buy two of everything. We've bought a playpen here and they bought a playpen there, we've got a cot here and they've got a cot there. Sometimes when our daughter asks if we could babysit, we encourage her to let the baby stay with them, because we see her more.

grandmother of one

180

My daughter's husband has three sisters and all of them have children – and those children depend quite a lot on that granny. She's got the hands full looking after the five of them. It's okay, I look after her son's children, so she doesn't have to worry much about that, and she can look after her daughters' children. It works out, it's balanced.

grandmother of four

They'd brought us together with the other grandparents, just so that we knew each other, because there wasn't a marriage at which we would meet. And later, when I was babysitting, the other grandparents were my back-up because they lived about ten minutes' walk away. So, they would be my first call if I needed extra help. I would like to be a bit more connected to them. I've occasionally met the other granddad and he's lovely.

grandmother of two

Or it may be to respect their particular needs:

When my daughter-in-law went into labour, my son phoned her mother, who lives in the north, and she got on the first plane and came down. We went out to the airport and took her straight to the hospital, but we didn't go in, we just let her. We just thought, it's *her* daughter – we went up later in the afternoon. We get on very well with them, they're very nice people.

grandmother of five

When my granddaughter was about six, the relationship of my son's partner and her own

181

mother started to improve. I think she made a concerted effort and now I see they're incredibly bonded – they live together half the week now. I was happy that the balance had been redressed. I thought it was right – I'd had a lot of time with my granddaughter and was so happy to have had that.

She and I talked about it quite a bit and she said, 'Well, you had the first six years, and now it's my turn.' And then my other son's twins were born, so my focus shifted, my attention then went over there.

grandmother of three

And there is the occasional cooperation for their respective children's benefit:

The other grandmother is an exceptional woman and she adores the grandchildren. She's very close to her son – she's always there and always available to the children. There's no competing on my end. I'm hugely grateful that she's there and involved. And she certainly doesn't want to take on any more load than she's already carrying – unlike me, she is still working, including long and difficult shifts. Her husband's been ill recently, so she's got a lot on her plate.

There was an incident when our children had a marital misunderstanding – she and I pulled together quite successfully. We picked the girls up and took them to my house. She said, 'If I go to my house, my son might be tempted to come home to me and I don't want him to do that. I want him to sit down with his wife until they've ironed out whatever it is.' So she stayed the night at my house with them.

The kids were asking 'Where's Mummy and Daddy? I said, 'Sometimes Mummy and Daddy just need to be Mummy and Daddy again because they don't get the chance much. And that's what Grannies and Nanas are for.' I hope we go on being a good double act. Because for me, it's a source of great pleasure.

grandmother of two

Sometimes, there can be difficulties over their different attitudes to child-rearing:

She's a lovely grandparent. I get on with her fairly well, although we're like chalk and cheese. But I find it frustrating to see my daughter having to put up with not having any control over her. She is very kind and generous, but imposes her own ideas. I am not allowed to feed those children any form of sugar, chocolate and so forth because my daughter doesn't want them to have these things.

But the mother-in-law, willy-nilly, 'Oh, I'm just giving them a treat or two.' Those children come out of her house bouncing off the walls, with a can of Coke.

grandmother of two

And some have relatively little contact, especially when they do not live near each other:

In my experience, there is often a cluster of involvement around the time when your children are getting married and when the first grandchildren arrive, you will see the in-laws quite often. And then, it gradually peters out. And of course they're all very dispersed. One of the other grandmothers lives not far away and we see her regularly, when there's a family lunch or a gathering, she will come.

grandmother of ten

My daughter-in-law's mother lives quite a distance away, so she's not competing with me, as it were. She's not offering the back-up that she would have welcomed from her own mother. She did come down to be with them after the birth and she was helpful, but they see much more of us than they see of her.

grandmother of two

Other children

The question then arises of how the birth of one or more grandchildren affects relationships with the other children, who might feel they get less attention from a busy grandmother. This does not seem to be a major issue. Often, grandmothers talk about how much their other children enjoy their siblings' children. In the case of young grandmothers, they sometimes have children not so different in age than their grandchildren:

My teenage son loves the baby. When he found out that his sister was expecting, he told everyone, 'I'm going to be an uncle' – he was really chuffed. And when the baby was born, he couldn't wait to get up and see her and he brought her a big balloon and a teddy bear. He is really good with her. He says he's going to teach her how to play his X-Box.

My other daughter is very good because she's done a childcare course and she knows at what age the baby should or shouldn't be doing things. She's not interested in having any kids yet – she likes to go on holidays, she likes to go out, she likes the job she's got.

grandmother of one

Older siblings also enjoy the new member of the family:

It's brought my other son absolute joy. He absolutely adores the little girl. We were always close – coming from a divorced background, I've always perhaps overcompensated with my sons and put everything of my life into them. He came yesterday for my granddaughter's birthday and, at Christmas time he's there playing with her all the time. He gets a lot of pleasure from her.

grandmother of one

The children love their uncle. He is a natural with children. He will sort-of inhabit their space and try to understand what's going on for them, from their point of view. I don't think he would feel resentful about my relationship with them, probably rather the opposite. And anyway, they love him. They'd rush to him if he appeared and rush away from me.

grandmother of two

In many ways, my son and I are closer now than we've ever been. He has a very nice girlfriend. Sometimes he'll come and stay for a week at a time. Funnily enough, my children fought like cat and dog when they were very small, but after they left home they both did the boomerang thing at the same time, both in their late 20s, coming back to live with me through a winter. It suited me quite well and they now have a very good adult relationship. He's a wonderful uncle.

grandmother of two

One sees the potential for competition, however:

If my daughter has a baby in the next year, I feel sure I will be needed, and then you are really torn. Because you have jealousy from other members of the family, who notice you're looking after one child, but what are you doing for theirs? And there's going to be less capacity, now that we're getting older. My husband has some health issues, which are taking up a bit of my time. I haven't got as much to give now, as I might have done when the first one was born.

grandmother of two

And sometimes, the presence of a grandchild has other effects on the siblings:

My youngest daughter's living with me now she says she's not having any kids until she's well into her 30s. Having all these here has shown her that it's not a picnic. That's fine. I want her to live her life. I had mine at 19, I don't really want that. They should have children after they've done what they want to do, at least see a bit of the world.

She minds if they go in her room and touch her stuff – they get in her make-up and what have you, spread it everywhere, and the little one will come out with her high heels on. It's like having little siblings. She makes sure she shuts her door now.

grandmother of six

We see a lot less of my other daughter, but that's not to do with the grandchildren – that's to do with her being dedicated to her job. She's done very well. We're always second, because she's always got other things going on. She is adamant that she will never have a family. She's said, 'I've watched my sister go through it and I love being an auntie and that's enough.' If she's happy, that's fine. I don't think people should have children willy-nilly.

grandmother of two

Grandfathers and their role
Last – but definitely not least – come the grandfathers. Many grandmothers comment that their husband or partner takes an interest in the grandchildren, but is somewhat less involved, in part because he is at work:

I had more time available, so if somebody needed picking up from a nursery, I would do the bulk of the childcare. My husband would always be there and close when he came home, but he was still full-time – that made a big difference. Alongside that, for the past seven years, he's been rather ill. He's ticking over quite well, but it's diminished his energy levels. But we talk about the family a lot.

grandmother of ten

My husband's always interested to know what happened, how did I spend my day with the baby – he wants a detailed account of everything, which I tell him. Sometimes I just give him the most interesting highlights – I don't always feel like repeating the day in my head anymore.

grandmother of one

When grandfathers do make an appearance, they seem to be the source of fun and possibly more spoiling:

My husband's more vigorous with them than I am, which is why it's good to have both of us there. Fighting on the floor with them, he will get them quite excited, rough and tumble. I am definitely the bottom-line person, the cook, the feeder – he is the swinging in the park or the rope ladders in the forest. He will do more adventurous stuff than I will, definitely more physical.

But if they're in a concert or something at school, we both try to go if we can. And if only one grandparent can go, we take it in turns.

grandmother of eleven

In our generation, the grandfather can be the fun figure. Grandmothers are often left to be more responsible for the children. I will go and take over and cook tea and that sort of thing. Her father is retired and lives on his own. Sometimes, she asks him to help with the children, but he doesn't like cooking the kids' tea. I said to my daughter, just buy a pizza. So Granddad is a real treat, because they get pizza.

grandmother of two

There was a point when Granddad turned up when our grandson was about one and he made a face and the boy was terrified. So, for the next few times, he didn't want Granddad. I smoothed that out and made it all right. Now, I sometimes feel a bit jealous of his pulling power – when he goes over there once a month, he is the star. He knows that, it's just how it is. I lose them to him.

grandmother of two

Or they may sometimes just be different in tone:

My little grandson will go in the bedroom in the morning and jump on the bed with the granddad. He'll get a big book and say, 'Now, read that to me.' And my husband will indulge him, read him a little bit and play. But I notice they don't talk that much. The boy knows his grandfather loves him, but he's more firm. And maybe he just knows that men just come and go, whereas the women are always around from morning to night.

grandmother of one

One Indian woman recounts the change over the generations, at least from her perspective:

In India, men don't do anything – they are just there to order people around. So my grandfather also just ordered things around. We used to go to him and say, 'Good-morning Dada,' and he would say, 'Good-morning, dear,' and that was about it. He didn't have much interaction with the grandchildren.

My father was different. He was absolutely over the moon having a granddaughter in the house. He was retired, so he would do everything with her. He would take her to the shops and buy her presents. In the evenings, because he was fond of gardens, he would hold her hand and take her round, and point out the flowers. He would play with her, but that's not the norm.

My husband's involved a lot. He's quite happy to. I don't drive, so he ferries me everywhere, and he's happy to do this for the sake of the kids. He plays cards with them, he plays board games, he does everything now. He likes to know what they are doing. He's told me many times, 'I've done far more for my grandchildren than I did for my children.' He'll go and sit outside her school waiting for her to come out. He feels bad that he didn't see our son grow up, because he was always abroad with business.

grandmother of two

Some divorced (or never married) grandmothers have new partners or husbands. Here, there is much less involvement with each other's grandchildren:

My current partner talks about being a grandfather. We do share experiences. I've met his grandchildren and he's met mine, but he's not very much part of our team. He likes them and they get along, but he and I have a separate life, separate from his family and separate from my family. I quite like that.

grandmother of two

Absent grandfathers

When the grandmother is divorced or separated from the grandfather, it seems to be particularly difficult for the grandfather to keep in touch:

> My ex-partner didn't have any involvement, because he's so far away and because, I suspect, the woman he's with guards him jealously. He's not the most responsible type of chap, but he's a very kind and loving man – he was wonderful bringing up our daughter when she was tiny. We barely see him.
>
> For a long time, our daughter got very upset that he didn't come down enough – she had to remind her daughter of who he was. Just recently, he's been down for a whole week – that was delightful and made up a lot of lost ground. We're hoping that he'll feel able to come down more.
>
> *grandmother of two*

> I think it differs if you are married grandparents. Divorced parents can be difficult to access. He lives outside London and he has taken her for a couple of days – he enjoys having her, but it's not as close as me, because I'm round the corner and I see her three or four times a week.
>
> *grandmother of one*

In some cases, the involvement with the absent grandfather is carefully fostered:

> I worked extremely hard to bring my ex-husband into a family situation. Both children were living at some distance and I urged them to make an

effort to keep in touch with their dad. Eventually, I invited him to join us at a family occasion and that broke the ice. And I gradually made sure that he was not left out on family occasions.

I think it's important that the children should see all of their grandparents. I don't want to get back together with my ex-husband, but I want the spokes of the family wheel to be there. They've got me there, they've got him there, they've got the other grandparents – all those spokes should be intact, to be used when needed.

grandmother of two

Grandmothers disagree on whether it is harder to be a grandparent when there is just one person:

It impacts quite a lot that I'm on my own. It's much easier with two of you. As a mother, you know how to deal with your children, you understand them, you've built up a kind of way of living. But, as a grandmother, you're coming into somebody else's way of living and it's much more exhausting. You're older and you have to cope with the children not the way you brought them up to behave, but the way they behave. If there are two of you, it's a lot easier.

grandmother of eight

My husband had died, so I could be there when I wanted – if I wanted them here for the weekend or a week if my daughter went away, I could have them. There was a time when they took the older one on holiday and I had the younger one. My son-in-law had a heart attack while they were away, so I had her for another three weeks. It's been good that I've been alone, because I've been able to concentrate on them without having to please a husband at the same time.

grandmother of two

Chapter 8
Looking Back and Looking Forward

Talking about their grandchildren reminds women of when their own children were small. This brings back a host of memories of the difficulties of parenting, coupled with comments on how much easier it is to be a grandmother than a mother. This, in turn, leads to thoughts on how they are part of a line, both genetically and in terms of family and cultural traditions. At the same time, they look to the future with a mixture of hope and concern. This chapter explores these issues.

Looking back on parenthood
The very fact of being a grandmother invariably makes a woman remember when her children were young.

The regrets
Probably the most common reaction, when looking back on their period as the parent of babies, small children and, indeed, teenagers, is how very difficult it all was. A number note how that they felt completely unprepared:

> I just regret that I wasn't as good at it as my children are. They do the research. My daughter reads it all up and they've got everything off the screen. Whereas I didn't know anybody who had a baby, anywhere. I never read a book, I never read a magazine article, I just sort of made it up as I went along.

> The only advice I got was from some rather worried health visitors who looked at me and my husband trying to raise this baby and thinking I'm clueless. I just hurtled into it and crash

landed, really. I'm very lucky that both of my girls have coped with being brought up in a rather hit and miss way.

grandmother of two

I don't think I was a good mother. I was an organised mother who gave them everything they needed, knew what was good for them, but I didn't just relax and sit with them hour after hour. When you're young, you're busy. You have responsibilities – you're filling your time with having to do things. I could've been a better mother by giving more time calmly to my children.

It changes with each child. With child number three, I remember coming back from a holiday thinking, thank God, now I can sit in our back garden and do nothing – just me and my baby. I didn't have that response with child number one.

grandmother of five

They often note the many things they got wrong, from the unimportant to the more significant:

I was a hard parent, partly because I had three close together. Some parents are quite happy for there to be a great din around them, but we both wanted it to be peaceful, so I'm afraid there were more stiff reprimands than my son and his wife ever give. And they are very tolerant, like seeing a child wanting to splash in a puddle. They've encouraged them to be very free, whereas I would say 'Don't go in that puddle!', because I was conscious of the amount of washing that that would engender.

I've often thought that if I were to do it all again, I wouldn't be so strict. You always wish you could have your time again – I would let them splash in puddles.

grandmother of two

I feel very guilty about letting my daughter go to boarding school. It was totally alien to my background – I only did it because I had this new husband, who wasn't her father and was never like a father to her, and he wanted her to go. I allowed it to happen and I never forgave myself for that. I still can't talk about it, because I cry when I talk about letting her go. But she doesn't seem to resent me for these things. I was always torn in two. My heart was always with her, but I was being sensible, having to keep the husband happy.

grandmother of two

I sometimes think I didn't pay enough attention to making sure they went to university and that sort of thing. I'm in two minds about that, because I don't think the whole world should feel that they have to go to university and there should be other things on offer. Perhaps that's the role that the husband normally takes – and he wasn't there to do it. But on the whole, I think it was good for them, that kind of freedom.

grandmother of eight

Making amends
Some grandmothers see their grandparenting as almost a means of making up for their deficiencies as mothers:

196

Looking back on bringing up the children, I wish that I had appreciated them more. And obviously, there's the chance with grandchildren to do just that. You can appreciate them and give time to them in a way that you couldn't when your own children were young. I was busy working, I had a career and all the rest. I think that's what I'd do differently if I had my time again. I'd appreciate them more.

grandmother of ten

I made mistakes as a mother, but I've tried to do better the second time around with the grandchildren. I was a single mum for a long time, it was hard. I'm sure I did things which were not done very well. I don't recommend it to anyone, being a single mum. Forty years ago, when women kind-of wrongly understood feminism, they thought they could do it on their own – but it's never to be recommended.

grandmother of two

But many feel there is nothing to feel bad about because they did not know better:

I don't have guilt feelings. Some of my friends say, 'I should've done this, I should've done that' – it's mainly those whose children haven't turned out to be quite stable. I just feel you do your best. I did my best as a parent and, after all, we were quite young – and you can't have regrets because what's done is done. You just have to get on with it.

grandmother of eleven

Of course, there are things that I've done in my life that I might have done differently with the benefit of hindsight. But my motto is 'Je ne regrette rien.' When my mother died suddenly when I was 17, the welfare officer from my Dad's firm said to me, 'I'm going to say something to you now that I hope will stay with you. There are two words that you don't use together – the first one's "if" and the second one is "only"'. There is nothing you can do.

You can't spend your whole life thinking if *only* I'd done this, if *only* such and such hadn't happened', so I don't do that.

grandmother of two

I feel that I didn't know any better when I was young, so why should I try to make amends? I don't have a guilty conscience. I would love that women would give up their guilty consciences, because if they knew any better then, they wouldn't have done whatever. I don't have any regrets. I am very realistic – there are times when I have really messed up with bringing up my children, but I didn't know any better.

grandmother of one

Proud mothers

Yet, despite all the soul-searching and the regrets, there is often a strong sense of pride in their child's upbringing. Sometimes, it is based on the amount of time they gave:

It does give me a sense of pride. I felt that they were my priority – they were fed well, they were looked after well, they always had a lovely, warm bed. I had plenty of time to sit and read with them. I just enjoyed having my children.

I think the poor mums of today – it's all rush, rush, rush. Rush to get out in the morning, rush to get back to work, rush to get home, rush to get the tea on the table. I'm not saying that's wrong. I'm just saying it's different.

grandmother of one

I loved being a mother. The only achievement in my life has been putting children on earth and making them who they are. And I feel I did it. I don't think my husband had as much to do with it as I did. It was all my own achievement.

grandmother of five

And sometimes, it relates to how things turned out:

I think I did quite a good job. They're nice people. My greatest achievement – I have two children and I like them both. Love is taken for granted, most people love their biological children. But they might not always like them.

grandmother of two

I do have some pride in my parenting. But more than that, what is so very good is that we have very good relationships now with our children and their partners. That's great. They have all formed long-term relationships, which is an indication that our role model was not all that bad. Everybody has had long marriages and I think that's an indication that they have seen the value of family.

grandmother of ten

I did a good job with them. I do praise myself many days. Because there's a house just across the street, the man's a drug dealer. I prayed morning, noon, and night that they didn't get mixed up with him. And they didn't. It's got even worse now – you'll see the kids going there to get their drugs.

grandmother of ten

Easier to be a grandmother than a mother

A very frequent comment is how much easier it is to be a grandparent than a parent. This is partly due to the lack of day-to-day responsibility:

One of the nice things about being a granny is that you don't have responsibilities. You don't carry that weight. You pass that to your children. If I do something wrong, I'm only a granny, I only see them very seldom. It's wonderful. I missed a lot of things when I was a mother because I was too busy.

grandmother of five

You know the parents are responsible and you're not, so it's a completely different relationship. It's not your fault if they go wrong. With my daughter, I can remember sitting on the bed when she was small, thinking, oh, what do I do now? We are completely responsible for this person. They're so tiny and vulnerable.

grandmother of two

You have more time to enjoy them. You're not having to teach them right from wrong, having to do the domestic side or the washing for them.

You notice more with your grandchildren, possibly because you have got the time.

When you're bringing up your own, you're doing everything. It's all your responsibility. But with your grandchildren, you notice all the little things that they do, their little ways, and they're just so joyous.

grandmother of one

And, as is often said, grandchildren get handed back at the end of the day:

The best thing about being a gran is you can treat them like your own, you can do whatever you want with them, but then you always hand them back. So I get all the joy, but come night time, he goes back to his mum.

grandmother of one

Even if they're being difficult, you've only got them for a limited period, and then you give them back! It's lovely. And the other thing is that you can have a slightly different relationship with them. I'm not as strict with them as I was with my own children. Because I feel that their parents can discipline them.

grandmother of eleven

It's easier to be a grandparent than it is to be a parent. I don't know if it's because you can give them back that you want to make the most of it when you've got them. It's hard to be a parent, because it doesn't come with a book. You just have to learn, don't you?

grandmother of eight

201

With grandchildren, there is more time to relax and enjoy the children:

> With the grandchildren, there are so many things I realise now which I could not give to my children when they were growing up. Time is the main factor. I was busy looking after my husband, looking after my house – you wanted to sit with them, but there was no time. You're so busy, sometimes you shout at them, you rush through everything.
>
> But when you have grandchildren, you are retired. You have more time to sit with them, to watch them growing, see their every moment – what they are doing, how they are laughing, what they want. You take the time out to give them those things – you're free now.
>
> *grandmother of four*

One grandmother feels it is something to do with being able to stand back if you need to:

> It's easier than parenting. Because you can withdraw if you need to. Whereas once you become parents, you're in it for the whole game, you can't withdraw. Once you've made love and realised that you've created a child, you have to give to that child.
>
> *grandmother of two*

Being part of a line

Seeing a family resemblance

Part of both looking back and looking forward for a grandmother is seeing herself or her children in the grandchildren. A few see traces of their family:

> I can't see myself, but my granddaughter looks ever so much like my son – both my sons, really, because they're quite alike. And he was a very easy child and she's got his nice, easy-going personality. It's quite rewarding.
>
> *grandmother of one*

> You wonder what's the baby going to look like, because there's all this lineage behind you, and somebody like the great-great-grandmother with bright red hair – is she going to come through in that child? My granddaughter looks very much like my mother's sister, who died when she was young. I'm very proud of the fact that I can trace my family back a thousand years. My parents had a researcher and we were able to trace them right back.
>
> *grandmother of three*

Some note how much different people see different likenesses:

> I saw a picture of my husband when he was four, and I said to my mother-in-law, 'Why have you got a black and white picture of my grandson?' And she said, 'It's not him – it's his father.' Some people say, 'This baby is exactly like his mother' and another will say, 'Oh, he is exactly

like the father' – I find it fascinating that people see different likenesses.

grandmother of five

A few see themselves in personal traits and characteristics, rather than looks:

She knows what she wants to do and she's doing it. In terms of her reports 'could do better' and her attitude of 'I'll do it later', that kind of thing – I can see myself.

grandmother of one

I've enjoyed seeing our family likenesses, I could see my son in certain behaviours in them. That is a kind of visceral, genetic thing – the selfish gene, seeing the next generation producing another generation, so it's been an added dimension which has been very enjoyable.

grandmother of two

Even a woman who was adopted feels there is some connection down the line:

I was brought up in a family with whom I had no genes in common. I was the cuckoo in the nest. I'm surprised sometimes at things that I see that are definite genetic family traits. When you're with the grandchildren, you're doing childish things with them and you think about yourself doing them, like climbing a tree or going on a trampoline. I remember doing those things, so my memory goes back to being that person and then I see the likenesses.

I think there is something wonderful about your child and your relationship with your child, which is unique. And it's unique with each grandchild. Because there's a part of you in them and even as an adopted child, I feel that I'm a part of those families that I was adopted by, not through nature, but through nurture.

grandmother of two

Some grandmothers simply like to see the sense of continuation:

It's very nice to have your genes going on. I sometimes miss my mum, who died not long ago. Before that, my grandmother went and before that my aunts and uncles. So, we all will go, but we are leaving behind a sample on this earth, in a way. And I think this is the way of life. Each one comes, dies off, leaves some sample behind. It's a circle of life.

grandmother of two

I'm not too concerned about the family line. I just feel happy that my daughter is a mum, because to have a child is fulfilling and completes a woman. And it's nice, the continuation. Not for lineage and you want your name to go on, but just continuation of life, of the next generation, that's all.

grandmother of one

But for one Hindu woman, the resemblance has enormous significance:

My husband was very unwell – and I lost him. And then, after one month or so, my daughter told me she was expecting twins. So it was first a very sad time and then she's giving me this news. We Hindus believe in reincarnation – the one who is gone is coming back. I said 'Daddy is coming back!' This father and daughter were very close to each other.

When the twins were born, I took the little girl in my hand and looked at her and she was smiling – and her smile was exactly my husband's smile. My son was standing there and I'm looking at him and saying, 'Do you see what I see?' He touched my shoulder, 'Yes, Mummy.' We both had the same feeling, that this little girl is smiling like Daddy.

And then, we are all just looking at each other and having the same thought – *he's back*! And that feeling is still there when I see her.

grandmother of four

Family traditions
In addition to a sense of the passage of genes, some grandmothers are very conscious of the passage of family traditions:

My grandmother was a good cook. She did things like meringues and fudge – all sorts of evil sweet things – and she wrote the recipes down. We have a family cookbook which my son has put together, including her recipes and others, which is online and available to all the family now. That's a way of passing a link of the families down.

Moreover, my grandfather was a metallurgist and, as a child, he started me off on collections of rocks. And even now I'm very interested in geology. In the same way, I started off nearly all the grandchildren with collections of rocks to foster this sort of interest. There are places where you can buy rocks and things and, for Christmas, I'll give them a little box with various labelled specimens.

grandmother of ten

When my daughter was first having the baby, I washed all the new clothes before I put them on the baby, so I knew that they were all clean and fresh. That's a thing that my nan did and my mum did, so it's come down from them.

grandmother of one

Some of these come from their particular cultural or religious background:

I think keeping kosher is important. Milk and meat are separate. The children's homes are all kosher It's a cultural heritage and it's a good way of life that I would like them to continue for their children. Our culture is also orientated to charitable giving. All my children are involved in charities and my two older grandchildren are now as well. That gives me pride that their parents have influenced them to want to give something back.

grandmother of eleven

Politeness is something we are brought up with in Barbados. You must always respect your elders, say good-morning, good-afternoon, whatever. And when you're sitting down to table, you must sit down until you've finished, you can't get up. I had a good upbringing and I passed it on to my kids. If they're rude, it's go to your room – no television, no nothing, just go.

grandmother of ten

In India, the grandmother is very important. My maternal grandmother doted on me because I was the only granddaughter. Although everybody in India wants sons, in our family they loved daughters. I was the only girl, so she was really over the moon. I got loads of jewellery as gifts – diamond stud earrings, necklaces and bangles. These are always passed on. I passed the studs on to my own daughter, she passed them to my niece and then they came back and were passed to my granddaughter. It gives such a good feeling that you're passing on something of your grandmother.

grandmother of two

And sometimes 'culture' is a local issue:

East End mothers are different – they're more hands-on. You can get some posh grandmothers that won't let the kids sit on the furniture or won't let the kids have a bit of chocolate in case they get dirty. Whereas in the East End, 'Oh, let them have a bit of chocolate – you can wash it out in the washing machine'. They're more easy-going. And very much more loving than people who have a baby for the sake of having a baby and get nannies in and then go back to work.

grandmother of one

The question of a child's name can also be important:

Mum didn't even see her granddaughter, which is a huge regret. I so much wanted to call my daughter after my mother, and then chose the name of somebody that I knew. And when she and her husband spontaneously decided to call their first girl after my mother, I was just overjoyed. It was a very special moment for me.

grandmother of two

One great-grandmother feels that traditions are important and is very regretful that she knows very little about her past:

To think two people could make all these children into one big family. I've made seven children and all these grandchildren. With grandchildren, in-laws, the grandchildren and their partners, I have a huge family! I feel proud. And they know me. They've got something to look back on when they get older and they have stories to pass on.

When you get older, you crave your past. I don't know my past and I haven't got any to pass on. I was 19 when my dad passed over, and 27 when my mum went. I wasn't old enough to think to question more.

When I'm gone, I want my family to be close and look after each other. I hope the grandchildren all keep close together and not forget where they come from. It's something about roots. If I could know my roots, I'd be a happier person.

grandmother of seven

Looking forward

Having grandchildren tends to make a woman look further into the future than ever before, as she wonders what life will be like for them.

Hopes for the future

Many grandmothers talk about their hopes for their grandchildren and the nature of their lives. Much of this concerns finding a good job and a good partner:

I hope and I pray that the grandchildren all get good jobs, don't get into trouble, make me proud of them and try to have a good life. I haven't had any problems with my children, and so far, they all got good jobs. I would like that for my grandchildren.

grandmother of ten

I hope that they have a happy life and are fulfilled – I know that's a bit cheesy, because nobody ever has the perfect life, but this is what I wish for them. And I hope my grandson who has particular problems is encouraged and helped, because he's an interesting little thing, but it's not going to be easy. Of course, you just wish them a lot of happiness – I know it's not going to be all roses, but that's my deepest wish.

grandmother of two

Not to mention having children:

I just want them to be happy and I don't care what they do – if they're a success or if they're not a success, I'll still be there. I'd also love them to have children because there's such a joy in having children. Fantastic. If I'm here, I'd love to see the great-grandchildren. Touch wood, my health is good.

grandmother of two

I keep praying that they will end up having beautiful families of their own. The oldest now is of the age. You have to support them with prayers, that God in his mercy will lead them to their rightful partner in life, because once you're able to find that, nothing will go wrong. I am hoping they will find a partner where they understand each other and make a blissful marriage, a happy home, and when they have their children, they'll know how to bring them up.

grandmother of three

Education is mentioned quite often:

Education is very important to us – if you have education, you can achieve what you want. I would like to see them doing well in life – well settled, with good jobs and good partners. It would break my heart if they ended up losing their way. We live in the hopes that our children will be doing as well, if not better, than us.

grandmother of two

I just hope that they can all train in something that will give them a job, and will have some financial security. It's very difficult these days.

For my grandson with problems, I just pray that he's mentally well, and if he can finish a degree and remain healthy, that would be enough for me.

grandmother of three

Sometimes, the hope centres on their inner lives:

I wish the earth for my grandchildren. I want them to have enough, but not too much. I hope they will love and feel close to people and will serve people, and be loved and be served by them. I would like them to be their own best friend - as well as to have best friends. I would hope that they will believe in something bigger than themselves, the Spirit or Love or Truth. Also curiosity and a thirst for understanding. And that they will have respect for all life, including their own.

grandmother of two

A lot of people say, 'What I want is for them to be happy', but I think, no, that isn't how the world works. I think 'interesting' is more to the point. And that they can cope.

grandmother of eight

I just hope he's going to be a good, upright young man. Honest, caring for others in a positive way, developing all his talents and skills. We believe you've got to play an active part in society, and in life. Get involved, do things – don't just sit. My motto has always been 'Be a participant in life, not a spectator.'

grandmother of one

And some talk about their future relationships in the family:

I hope the grandchildren will get on with each other. I think siblings getting on with each other is tremendously important in later life. You're going to need support in life's troubles. I have good relationships with my sisters and I'm conscious of how important that is.

grandmother of two

I hope my new grandson will have a loving and empathic relationship with his parents, wanting to please his mother, but also able to grow into independence. I hope she will show him loving warmth and affection, praising and valuing him – and that they enjoy being together. I also hope she will set up firm boundaries so that he feels safe, but will move them when she realises they don't work!

grandmother of one

A few, with grandchildren who are babies or toddlers, consider the nature of their relationship with the grandchildren in the immediate or longer term:

I hope we'll be really good pals, that she'll be able to confide in me. Little things that happen at school, if she's got a problem – maybe it's easier to talk to a nanny than to talk to your mum and dad. I hope she'll be able to feel free to talk to me like that.

grandmother of one

I've made a bit of a calculation – when I am 68, my grandson will be 10. I will still have a lot of time and energy. I don't know what the music style will be in ten years' time, but if I'm alive, I would go with him. I love to imagine taking him to scouts or collecting him from birthday parties, inviting his friends round and making something nice for them. And then, I think, we will have a good bond and I'd love to give him a good memory of his grandmother.

grandmother of one

I'm looking forward to going on holidays with him. And taking him out to parks. Taking him to school and picking him up. I just hope that when he does grow up, I'll be in a better financial situation where he could come to me and say, 'Nana can you buy me this?'

grandmother of one

Concerns for the future

Grandmothers can be very alert to the many difficulties of the modern world. They speak eloquently about their concerns. Some of these pertain to the immediate world around their grandchildren, especially those who live in poorer areas, and its potential impact on their lives:

It is changing a lot round here. When we were young, we could play out in the streets and be safe. There's just too much drugs on the street, too much crime, too much knifing, too much racial tension. I want my granddaughter to go to a nice school where she's going to be taught and not bullied. And you never heard of TB years ago, now it's rife around here. There's a hell of a lot more to worry about now.

grandmother of one

All this violence that's going on in the streets today. It's just the fear of my grandson getting caught up in gangs and all that. He does a lot of evening activities to steer him from the streets. In my time, you'd play in the streets, I used to be out all day. But you couldn't do that now. If it's like this now, what's it going to be when the little one is a teenager?

grandmother of one

They don't have the freedom that we had as children. We'd be out all day – you only went in when you got hungry. I can remember when I was 9 or 10, getting on a red bus rover in the school holidays and going all over London. Now, the kids are mainly indoors on their computers – life's changed. I think it's a shame.

grandmother of six

Some take a longer term view, with a concern that it may be difficult to find a satisfying job – or any job at all:

I have concerns about how it's become difficult to find jobs that are really rewarding, if at all. And the cost of housing. Whereas we – and even our children – could move out fairly early on and be independent, now people are staying home far, far, too long because they can't afford to move out – and that's a terrible turn of events.

grandmother of ten

I don't want my kids to have any more children, because it's so hard now. My granddaughter can't get a job. It hurts, because there's lots of things that I can't afford, her mum can't afford, so she has to do without. Having money to go to the shop or go for a meal with her friends – she can't do all that. I don't want them to get kids unless they've got a career, got a bit of money, have somewhere nice, a home to put them in and things like that.

grandmother of ten

Some are worried about the nature of modern society:

I just think the world that they're growing up in is so much harder than what we knew. I grew up in the '50s, '60s – we played outside, we interacted with other children. We all just followed whatever we were going to be. We felt free. My concern is the children are growing up without much interaction with other human beings. I am a bit scared about the technology.

grandmother of one

People are investing too much in material wealth. You turn on the radio and just keep hearing about growth – growth isn't what we need, not money growth. We don't need to be forever having more things. We need to become more aware of the things that matter and sharing community with people and having less things. Spending money on more and more up-to-the-minute technological things and on just anything you feel you want – it's not the way to live.

grandmother of two

Quite a lot of my generation are worried about what sort of world we are leaving for our children and grandchildren. Surely we didn't mean it to be so difficult for them to buy or rent a home or get a job with reasonable hours. Or to have to live without the security of public services we used to know. How can it be that we don't want our grandchildren to go to university because it will saddle them with crippling debt?

Then there's war and pharmaceuticals and everywhere a mess of motor traffic, not to mention the state of the climate. We all worry about different things. How did we get it so wrong for them?

grandmother of two

And some worry about the long term of the planet:

The whole state of the world terrifies me – the arms race, the wars all over the place, global warming, the way we don't seem to learn anything and we never seem to get any better. That's always been the same, and I suppose grandparents have always worried about that. But I do worry about the world that they're going to have to cope with.

grandmother of eight

I don't watch the news. If I thought about it, I'd be very worried for what our legacy is to them. My son is very environmentally conscious, he says that my generation destroyed the planet and that his generation is trying to do their best to put it back together again.

grandmother of two

I am worried about the future. The climate is changing and we're going to be overcome with floods and land is going to disappear. Where are they going to live? Are they going to be able to survive? And, where it's a nuclear age, are they overdoing it? I do worry that the world's going to tilt with so many people on it, is it going to become too heavy? I do worry that the world is not going to last.

grandmother of seven

Being a burden

For older grandmothers, looking forward also means thinking about reaching the end of their lives. A big issue is being a burden on the family:

All of us who are growing older are worried about how much of a burden we may be later on to the family. I don't know anybody who doesn't worry about that. The last thing I want to do is tie up my daughter or have any of her children have to look after me. They've already had quite enough in their lives of looking after people who can't cope.

And living with them would be a great mistake. We have a very good relationship at the moment, but that would totally change. I will become a very crabby old person when I can't do things any more.

grandmother of eight

I take each day as it comes. I say to my children that I don't want to see the day when I have fallen ill so that they have to look after me. I don't talk much about it, but sometimes I say to them 'If I become disabled, just kill me.' I don't want to be a burden on anyone. I just wouldn't want to find that I'm not able to do anything and they have to do it for me.

grandmother of four

I don't want anyone to have to look after me. I'm terribly independent. I never go to the doctor. I've lived here for 30 years and I've been about four times. A new doctor phoned me up this winter and said she'd like me to come in and see her. The moment I made the appointment, I felt ill!

I never tell my daughter if I have a bad cold, I just stay in. I don't want anyone fussing about me. The rest of the family are the hypochondriacs. They're always at the doctor's, my grandchildren, my daughter, and my son-in-law.

grandmother of two

One woman notes that had just seen an example of this situation and it made her even more aware of the issue:

I've just spent three days staying with a 92-year-old and I don't want to be in her situation. She does have a reasonable quality of life, but she's becoming physically very infirm and she's fighting what she sees as the control that her sons and daughters-in-law have over her.

A lot of my generation are determined that we're not going to be physical wrecks. If it came to it, we possibly would do something about it – we don't generally have religion and don't believe in an afterlife.

grandmother of two

Some say that they make a bit of a joke about the issue:

I say, 'When I'm old, you'll have to come and do this for me...' They shriek with laughter, 'Oh, you'll never get old, Granny, you'll never get old.' When my husband was seriously ill and there was a chance that he wouldn't live too long, we had to explain to the older ones that Grandpa had this cancer and he might not survive. So they've already faced the potential loss of a grandparent – and this is part of life.

grandmother of ten

My granddaughter's already told me that when I get sick, it'll be her mother who looks after me. I'm sure she was joking, but when my mum was getting older, she had a knee replacement. My daughter was practical and then the granddaughter sweeps in as the favourite – the cheer-er up-er. She's got it into her head that the next generation is the one who looks after the sick person and the one below is the one who swoops in and cheers them all up. She's said that's what she'll be.

grandmother of one

And some begin to plan for it:

I don't worry about my own passing, but I worry about my husband, he already has bad health. I keep telling him that we should downsize and move near our daughter. I have three friends who are very ill. They have children, and one of the friends has got daughters living on the same street and they are giving them a lot of support. So, I keep saying 'We have to start preparing ourselves. We are healthy today, but we don't know what lies for us ahead.'

grandmother of two

One grandmother, housebound with some of her family living upstairs, although having her physical needs looked after, already feels like an emotional burden:

My family doesn't come to visit me. I ring them up and ask them to come, but they don't – or they change the date and then don't come again. It is the tradition of 'It doesn't really matter, it's only an old woman.' I had some relations who came for half an hour and said they'd come again, but they didn't.

Time moves in a different way for them. After they've been, 'Oh, it was so nice, I'll come again next week.' It's genuinely meant. But, next week, they ring and say they can't make it – they're busy, they've got things to do. Whereas for me, time is different. The meaning of time changes with old age – it goes much faster. I have to ask them again and again – in fact, it's become a joke, 'I'm not dead yet, are you coming to see me?'

My large old family house is derelict now, it's my tragedy. That house, which we built and furnished and we did everything with, is completely derelict, nobody's looking after it. My husband left me and I wasn't well – I survived in the house for about four years and then I came here. And nobody's doing anything about it, we're afraid to touch it. It's a metaphor – that derelict house is a metaphor of me.

grandmother of five

The fragility of life
Not surprisingly, older women start to think about the fact that their life is not endless:

In life, there's death. If I'm here, I'm here. At the age of 17, my life went into a black hole because my mother was killed in a car accident. So I don't expect anyone to be here tomorrow. Will I be here? Will anybody we know be here?

I grew up in a huge family. You had christenings, confirmations, weddings, funerals. People die, it's part of life. My favourite uncle dropped down dead in his forties – it was very distressing, but this is part of life and you have to deal with it. Maybe I'll get to see my grandchildren grow up, it'd be very nice.

grandmother of two

I hope I'll have the energy to continue for many years, but I know realistically, I'm unlikely to see the newest grandchild married. You have to be realistic about it. There's a slight sadness, but I feel we have a lot of pleasurable things to look forward to in the meantime. I just hope to keep my health and strength and to be able to get out and about.

grandmother of eleven

Such concerns may be particularly vivid for those in ill health:

I'm not in good health, I've got emphysema and bad arthritis, but I don't worry. When my time's up, it's up – and I've had a good life with them. I think it worries them more than me. I started smoking again and they say, 'Oh, Mum, you shouldn't' and I think to myself, what do you mean, I shouldn't? If I'm miserable, then I'd rather be happy and die happy, than give up smoking and be miserable.

grandmother of eight

There's nothing left for me now, only the box. I don't let it bother me, I just take each day as it comes. I give God thanks that I'm still breathing and I get on with it. Whatever is to be, will be. I'm just praying that when the time comes, I don't suffer too much. I don't want my children to be worried about me, I'd just like to be quick. But I'm not looking to my kids for anything. All I want is for them to look after themselves – I don't want anything from them.

grandmother of ten

A few discuss this, either directly or casually, with their grandchildren:

Occasionally, I talk to them about when I'm dead and gone. I was teaching my granddaughter to cook something and she found it difficult. I said she would do fine, it's only because I cook the same thing every day, so 'You will do the same and when I'm dead and gone, you will remember my words.' And sometimes I suggest to my grandson, who also likes to cook, why doesn't he write the recipes down. 'You'll remember them and then when I'm dead, you'll say, oh, these were Nani's recipes.'

grandmother of two

One granddaughter said, 'Grannies die and then they come back again.' I said, 'No, they don't come back again. They go up in the clouds and keep an eye on you, to keep you safe always. So, if the ball goes in the road, they remind you that you mustn't run after that ball.' And, of course, I told a lie.

grandmother of five

The occasional grandmother feels that this may be a problem for the grandchildren:

I worry about being very close to them, because I'm not going to last forever. When I go, will they do all right? I fear that they'd miss their granny because it was too strong a part of their lives. If you're not there, you leave a very big gap. That's the only thing that worries me slightly. I'd be glad if they weaned off a bit.

grandmother of two

Chapter 9
Reflections on Being A Grandmother

Throughout these chapters, grandmothers have offered many reflections on their experiences of being a grandmother and the emotions associated with it. Here, a few final thoughts are offered.

Finding the right balance

An underlying issue for grandmothers is finding the right balance between attending to their own lives and to those of their children and grandchildren. This can be difficult for a variety of reasons and is expressed in a number of ways.

Keeping the right distance

A major concern here is the need to avoid interfering too much in the lives of their children and grandchildren:

> One very difficult thing is to give up being the mother – in terms of being in control, doing the organising and being the person who is the centre of attention. It's very hard to know when to get involved and when to stay away. I do think grandmothers often make the mistake of trying to interfere. Trying to be either too important or too influential. It's what they're used to being – the head of the family.

> That's a difficult thing to give up. They can make the mistake of trying to be more important than the parents, wanting to be loved more. I've never been in that position, so that's never cropped up.

It's taken me quite a long time to let everything go and just be a person. But I have got on much better with my daughter since I found out how to do it – and she and I are now very good friends. We phone each other, we go out together to galleries and things.

grandmother of eight

It's a bad grandmother who undermines the security of the family – telling the children that you're right and they're wrong. That's just not on – if you're going to interfere in the wrong way, the family are probably better off without you. There's a lot to be said for knowing when to withdraw. You mustn't become dependent or feed off other people's lives. You have to have your own life very independently.

grandmother of two

A good nan, in my eyes, would be hands-on if they need your help, but not pushy. I wouldn't push myself on them if they didn't want me to. Some people can just take over, not listening to what the daughter's saying. I don't really take over, I let my daughter do things as she wants, but I do advise her.

grandmother of six

Having their own life
Many grandmothers have a natural wish to do other things for themselves and do not want the role of grandmother to dominate their lives. This may be a question of their own work or their own time with their husband or partner:

My husband and I don't get as much time as we'd like with one another. When our daughter's not here, we tend to use the time to catch up with 'just us'. We go out for something to eat, or pop round to his brother for a drink – it's just time spent like that.

My husband's been seriously ill – that did have a big impact on my life. When we first found out, I thought if anything was to happen to him, I'd be lost. He's not only my husband, he's my friend – he's everything.

grandmother of one

I'm just trying to live my life in the way that I'd like to live it. I'm a bit unusual because I'm still working, although I am well over retirement age. I decided about two years ago that I wasn't going to write any more books, but I still do bits and pieces. And I sing and I'm learning how to etch and I'm learning French, so there's a lot going on.

The grandchildren are not the only thing in my life, I don't rely on them as being the only thing that is meaningful.

grandmother of eight

I do a lot less voluntary work than I used to, because I try to prioritise the grandchildren if I'm needed. But you do need your own life. I believe that everybody has to have their own bit of independence and their own life. Your children have their lives. You can't help but take an interest and feel a pride, but you need your *own* interests. I think it's terrible to try to live your life through your children or your grandchildren.

grandmother of eleven

Some even take a change of direction:

About five years ago, my daughter said to me 'All your life, you've been thinking of me and my children – you've done enough, why don't you think of yourself?' And it dawned on me that they're not babies anymore. So I went to do a training for the Ministry and I became a pastor. I also try to write. My passion is to write more about the Word of God. That's my calling and if I can write ten books from the Bible, that would be awesome.

grandmother of three

We're all living longer. There's so much on offer in the world, so you want to enjoy life, do things that you never got a chance to do. I started a creative writing group for Muslim women. For some reason – culture, religion – they're very difficult to get out of the house. I targeted women over 40 whose children were a bit grown up and they were sitting at home not doing much. Most of them are grandmothers.

I was amazed by these ladies – they were all educated, but they put their degrees up on the wall when they got married and just looked after their husbands and children and forgot about themselves. Now, they're gaining the confidence to set boundaries, so they have time for themselves.

grandmother of one

And it can be a constant juggling act, trying to find the right boundaries:

I don't organise my life around them. I remember my partner saying, 'Now that you're retired, you can pick the boy up from school' and I thought, no, this is *my* time. If they tell me that he needs to be picked up, I certainly will. But I didn't want something to become a routine where I would *have* to do it, as a matter of expectations.

grandmother of two

It's not the main focus of our life – it's *a* focus. We carry on doing the things we are doing anyway in retirement, keeping up with our friends and relations and going away for weekends. We're not thinking, oh, we can't go away for that weekend because we need to see the grandchildren.

grandmother of two

Of course, they do not always feel that they get the balance right:

I looked after the children while my husband, my son and daughter-in-law went off to the Olympics. I had thought that would be fine, because I'm not that interested in sport. But I got really interested in what was going on, because of the lovely way the volunteers were helping and that 'feel-good' factor. I never got into the big Olympic stadium, and then I felt like Cinderella not going to the ball. But it was my own fault. Fortunately, most of the time, I don't feel taken advantage of.

grandmother of two

Moving to be near the family

In addition, there is the vexed issue of whether grandparents should move to be near their children or grandchildren. Many are very clear that they want to maintain their independence:

My son is always saying he wants to take me with him wherever he goes. But I like my home. I like my own space. I drive, so wherever they go, I can go. I like to do what I want when I want to do it and not have to consider other people. Of course, if they left the country, it would break my heart.

grandmother of eight

We've got a lot of Sikh families around here and often you'll get multi-generations all living together. I don't think I could put up with that – and I wouldn't expect my children to do so. I wouldn't have found it easy to have had my mother or mother-in-law living with me. Everyone's entitled to a little bit of privacy, including the grandmother.

I wouldn't move to follow the children. I don't believe in trying to step into their lives. It could create friction and you need your independence as long as you can have it. My interests are not their interests. I do know grandparents who move in with the children, but you've got to be very, very tolerant for that to happen.

grandmother of eleven

I go on the train to my daughter's every other week. I stay there for three days, I've got my own room there. But I like where I live. And I think it's their life – they don't need me in their life like that. I wouldn't want to live with them – I like to help, but I like to have my own life as well. Otherwise, they might just take over, telling me what to do and all that.

grandmother of six

Some comment that it might be fruitless to move to be near their children, because there would be no certainty that they would stay put:

I don't see any point in moving to be near the children, because they might easily move. These days, anybody can go and live anywhere. So that wouldn't make a lot of sense – and it might make them feel they had to stay where they were. So, I would go and visit them wherever they are. But, I have my own life and my own friends and they are important to me as well.

grandmother of eight

For those living near their children, discussions of a hypothetical move away can be painful:

If they went up to Scotland to be near her family, I'd be heartbroken. I can't really bear to think about it. My saving grace is that my son's business is in London, so for the foreseeable future, I see them being nearby. I don't think I would move if they did, because I've got my other son here, as well as lots of friends. Let's hope it never crops up.

You need to be near if you're going to be a proper part of their life. I know the other grandmother loves the child, but you don't have the same relationship from a distance. They don't see her on a day-to-day basis. She's very close to me, but if she lived far away, it would probably be different.

grandmother of one

My daughter stays with us most of the time and I take care of the baby. We love having them. They want to get their own place – they would prefer something close by, but they can't afford to buy and the rent around here is too high. We will really miss her, because the baby always wakes up happy, she shouts 'Nan' and "Granddad' first thing. The house will feel empty.

grandmother of one

And some have faced it already:

When they moved to Australia, it was hard. But my children grew up with no grandparents around because they all lived elsewhere, so it's in our family. I suppose, in the back of my mind, it was inevitable that one of them might move, just as we had done, away from our home countries.

My daughter-in-law wanted to go back north where she is from and they did go back up there. The day they left was horrible. I never felt bitter or anything – it's what I did to my parents and my husband did this to his parents – any argument would be very hypocritical.

grandmother of five

One grandmother notes that she recently moved to be near her grandchildren, but it wasn't easy:

I was ready to leave and it's not very far away from where I was. It's not certain that they will always stay here when the kids leave primary school. I had to think about what it meant if I was buying a house that I was going to live in forever. As it happens, I know people here. If I'm going to live on my own, this is probably as good a place as any.

grandmother of two

In great contrast, some have lived together all or most of their lives. There are often mixed feelings about this:

I have two of my children living here. Sometimes it's hard, like when they don't help me to do anything. I do all the cleaning. I cook during the week, my daughter's supposed to cook on weekends, but she doesn't. My son works late, he needs a meal when he gets home, so I get on with it. I think if I had a husband, he would speak up and they wouldn't take so many liberties with me, but they know I'm on my own. I get a bit tired.

grandmother of ten

It's nice having them all here because I've got company. When you've got young children around you, it keeps you younger. It keeps you up with the kids – you know a little bit of what's going on out there, instead of sitting back in an armchair and not doing anything.

But there are disadvantages. Normally, you can give the grandchildren back at the end of the day, but if they're living with you, you can't do that. When they were younger. I'd go to my room, close my door and say, 'I'm having five minutes, I don't want anyone in.' Now they're near adults, if they've got anything on their mind, like girlfriends or things, if they feel unable to talk to their mum, they'll come in and speak to me.

grandmother of seven

Sometimes I wish they would always stay here because of my grandchildren. I love having them here. I don't like having my daughter that much because she creates a lot of work for me, but I love *them* around. I wouldn't want them without her, because I couldn't handle that. So I've got to have *her* with *them*! They may be going soon in any case. I've told her, when he gets older, just send them to me. I would love to do things with them.

grandmother of two

In one case, there are four generations living together:

I lived with my mum off and on for years and I still am. It did cause problems for my son, because he had two people telling him what to do. He used to play us both up to get what he wanted. My little granddaughter went through a stage of drawing on the wall. I'd clean it, and say, 'We won't tell Great-Nanny, because she'd tell us both off.' I'm the one who gets them out of trouble from her. But my mum's got the last word. I'm still a child, because it's hard to take a role as a mother when you're living with your mother.

grandmother of two

The status of grandmothers
It is often argued that older women are not valued in modern society and, by extension, there is less respect given to grandmothers than in more traditional times. These grandmothers have complex views on this subject.

Feeling valued
A number of grandmothers do feel that they are respected and valued by their grown up children:

I know my son appreciates me. He always thanks me for doing things. Just the thank-you is enough. You don't want them kissing your feet, but it's nice being appreciated and valued. I think some people take advantage of their parents, with regard to grandparenting duties, but I'm lucky. Mine doesn't.

grandmother of one

I do get recognition. When I had such terrible problems with one son, I was in much despair, feeling I must have done something very wrong. My other son said this wonderful thing to me, 'Mum, so many of my values now – and how I'm bringing up my daughter – are what I've learnt from being your son.' And my granddaughter is very protective of me. She's just coming out of that awkward phase and always gives me big hugs and looks at me very directly – I feel that's very nice.

grandmother of three

And one daughter speaks directly about her own respect for her living mother, the great grandmother of her grandchildren:

My Mum was more or less a one-parent family, because what did Daddy contribute? I'm proud of my mum and so should every one of my brothers and sisters and her grandchildren be. The legacy should live on. She's brought up seven children and none of us are mass murderers or rapists or anything bad. She's done really well and she needs a pat on the back, because she's been a brilliant mother and grandmother and great-grandmother.

grandmother of two

On the other hand, a number do not feel properly valued at all by their children, whether for themselves or for their ability to contribute meaningfully to the grandchildren:

We can give a lot to the children – we've got a lot of experience and we did bring up our own children – but it's taken for granted. Young people just see the mum as a babysitter. When I'm at work, it's ok, the baby's with mum! I don't think they *value* the grandmother that much.

It's not just in our Muslim culture – I've seen it with English grandparents, with Jewish grandparents. I've heard them all talk about how the young will use the mums, but they don't really learn from them on how to bring their children up.

grandmother of one

Sometimes I don't feel that I am valued. I don't think that my kids do enough for me. If I didn't ask my son to do the lawn for me, he wouldn't do it. He's going to be 50 this year and I still have to ask – I don't think that's right. The same with the grandchildren. I get a card on Mother's Day. I might get a bunch of flowers, but that's about it. One daughter is the only one that would think about taking me out for a meal on my birthday or anything like that.

grandmother of ten

In the past, grandmothers were made use of. Now, they're put away, locked up in a room. They feel 'We have to keep an eye on you, make sure the doctor comes, the tests have been done' and so on, but if they've done all that, they've done their job and can enjoy themselves.

I don't think there is a place for a granny in society today. I can do very little because of my heart, I'm stuck within two rooms. I do keep myself busy, but it's not being part of a social structure. I can see all the grannies locked up in different rooms in all the houses in the world.

grandmother of five

When it comes to the grandchildren, grandmothers tend to feel appreciated, but in different ways depending on their age:

I think the four-year-old likes me. He knows I'm an adult who is obviously very fond of him, and he gets something from that. And the toddler is very affectionate – he clearly knows who we are, pats the chair to get you to sit down, brings a book and climbs on your lap – very relaxed. They certainly bound to the door when we go there.

grandmother of two

I think my teenage granddaughter is quite proud of me. I'm younger than some of the friends' parents and she's said that some of them think I'm a 'groovy' granny. In fact initially, they were amazed that I was a granny at all – I think she kind of enjoys that.

grandmother of one

My grandchildren are all adults and they seem to think of me in a warm kind of way. Somebody they're pleased to come to see. But I don't have the close relationship with them that some grandmothers have, who have spent a lot of time looking after them when they're young.

One thing I like is the pleasure I see in them when they see me, which means I'm giving them something they enjoy. When I go round to my daughter's, for example, the face of my granddaughter – who's a very sophisticated 20-year-old – lights up. That gives me huge pleasure.

grandmother of eight

But sometimes, relations are more complicated:

Because I turn up once a week, I'm like part of the furniture. I'm a bit taken for granted. It's good in a way, because I'm so close to them. It used to be that their mother would come home from work and there would be a very deliberate turning away from me, as though it was my fault that Mummy wasn't there before. And she wouldn't kiss me good-bye. It was quite wounding. I can't really plumb the depths of how much I minded about that. But now it's changed.

grandmother of two

I think my teenage granddaughter feels sorry for me. She doesn't want me to be on my own. And now that I've been in this new relationship for six months, I think she's relieved that I have somebody, another person in my generation who is maybe going to look out for me. She's says she wants to meet him and I'm happy about that.

grandmother of three

One grandmother feels her grandchildren give respect in their own way:

My granddaughters are mad about me – as I am about them. We have this fantastic relationship – please God, it never changes. Sometimes, they'll say something that is very rude and if I look funny, they'll say, 'Do you want us to treat you like a grandma, with proper respect?' and I say, 'No, carry on.' They all know my background – show business, flirty and all that – but that's our relationship, there's no sitting on being polite.

grandmother of two

A great-grandmother says it can be difficult for her:

> I expect respect from my grandchildren and great-grandchildren. I'd like them to realise that maybe I've only got ten more years, so make the most of me while I'm here. Come and visit me more, do more things together. My children are grandparents themselves, and of course the grandchildren are going to go to their parents first. We're shelved in a way, put on the shelf. Their life is wrapped up in the 'now'. I've got a young outlook, but I'm not young.
>
> ***grandmother of seven***

Being a matriarch

Grandmothers generally find themselves at the top of a family tree. This raises the question of whether they see themselves as a sort of matriarch. Some clearly do:

> I do feel that I am a matriarch – I am at the centre of it all. My nephew just got married and his new wife told my daughter 'He's told me about everybody and he said that everything happens around your mum – she has all the parties and she has all the opinions about everyone.' I just always have been. I got impatient with the others who didn't want to do anything, so I just took over from an early age. I'd have all the gatherings – the Eids and the Ramadan – I had the energy and the good heart and everything to do it.
>
> ***grandmother of one***

> When my mother was alive, she was definitely the matriarch. She was a very strong character, who lived to be 96. The children all respected

her opinion – even if they didn't, she would still give it. I believe I do, too, in a way.

My husband and I always feel great pride when we sit at the table and see all the family sitting round, happy to be together. We think about my father and how proud he would've been, because he went many years without children and his whole life was his children.

grandmother of eleven

I sort-of feel like a matriarch. I do think that they see me as somebody who knows how to 'be'. I think that is important. But it's very difficult. I know a lot of grandparents – their *all* is in the grandchildren.

I feel my grandchildren are a part of the texture of my life and I hope that I'm part of the texture of theirs, but I'm not the key figure for any of them. I feel that they're woven into my life in a way that is important, of course, because every thread woven into a life is important.

grandmother of eight

A great-grandmother feels this even more strongly:

I'm the matriarch – it's my family, I'm the eldest. There's about twenty-two of us, with the grandchildren and great-grandchildren. My children are off in their own lives in different places, I don't see a lot of them now. We get in contact birthdays, Mother's Day, Christmas. I remember some birthdays, but I have to be reminded of other grandchildren. But Christmas, there's always a present. I just buy the great-grandchildren mostly. And those who are close.

grandmother of seven

An Armenian grandmother feels it is part of her culture:

As a nation, as a culture, we Armenians are a very matriarchal society. Woman have a very important role in the family – big respect – and basically, the woman is the ruler of the house. The man is only the earner, the provider. It fits with my age and position in life. It is the next level of 'becoming whole' – to me, it's like a spiritual enlightenment.

I have always felt in need of becoming a grandmother. It's the way nature works. My sister hasn't got any children, but I see her as a grandmother in a different way. It is not necessary to have a physical grandchild to become a grandmother. It is a stage in a woman's maturity.

grandmother of three

And one woman points out the contrast with grandfathers:

Grandfathers have not given birth – their bodies aren't so involved. There's the age-old feeling of the woman doing the feeding and helping the bodies to grow and the minds to grow. It's not Father Earth, it's Mother Earth – something about Earth Mother and the grandmother is part of that too. So the matriarch is something about

Mother Earth and helping them to grow, Grandmother Earth.

grandmother of two

But others clearly do not see themselves in this light:

I'm not a matriarch. I'd quite like to be, but I'm not. The other nanny is a matriarch. She's got two daughters. There are photos of the three generations. Nanny in her wedding dress, her other daughter in her wedding dress (my daughter-in-law hasn't got one because she didn't get married), and that daughter's eldest daughter in her first communion dress. So, there are these women in white – and a photograph of the female line. Females are very strong in that family.

I quite like the idea of matriarchies, valuing the woman's role – it's female wisdom and female caring, the looking after people, the nurturing of the mothering and the grandmothering. Whereas the father has the 'protect and provide' role, still, even though women are going out to work.

grandmother of one

I don't have that power. This generation growing up doesn't need a matriarch. Life has changed so much. I think that's gone out. One niece came in the other day, age 17, looking gloriously attractive. I said, 'I'm looking to see how many young men are following you through the door!' And she said, 'To dress does not mean "yes".' These are the little empowering things they are being given.

grandmother of five

An Indian grandmother feels that the reverse is the case:

> We are more patriarch. My husband is the authority in the household, so whatever happens here, it always goes through my husband. I don't assert, I don't say, 'This has got to be done.' If my son rings and asks if we would like to go for a meal, I'll tell him, 'When Papa wakes up, I'll ask him, and if it's okay, I'll give you a call back.' And if he doesn't want to go, I don't go. That's my upbringing.
>
> ***grandmother of two***

Wisdom

Sometimes, older people are considered the source of wisdom. Some grandmothers feel that they are:

> On the spiritual level, being a grandmother allows you to commune with the feminine aspect of you that is wiser, stronger, the crone. It's contact with the spirit of the Big Mother and that is absolutely empowering. Maybe I have always been connected to that, because of my belief system.

> When my daughter had her baby, people started saying, oh, you are now a grandmother, grandma, nan, different names – at first, it seemed a bit patronising. But then I realised, they are reminding me of my initiation. And I said, 'Oh, yes, I *am*, thank you.' I became aware that is such an empowering place to be.
>
> ***grandmother of one***

When my daughter-in-law became pregnant, I decided to give up work so that I would have more time to spend with this grandchild and any others. I wanted to make sure that I had room for them. It's put me into the next phase of life – of being the crone, the older woman having the grandmother wisdom, caring for other people as an older person.

They were in my heart when they were tiny. I was old and they were young and I could pass on wisdom – or at least love – to them. It is built into my bones, in the third stage of life, to nurture young ones, especially the ones I have an unbroken blood link with.

grandmother of two

It probably makes you a lot wiser than you were before. You have to be thinking a lot about the way people are and what your particular people are. By the time you become a grandmother, you have a much wider experience and view of things. If you use that, you can get to understand people a bit better.

grandmother of eight

One suggests it comes from God:

God gave me three beautiful grandchildren, not because I deserve them, but because He wanted me to lead them, to guide them until they become adults and to bring them up in the way of the Lord. Show them the right thing in life and when they are trying to deviate, bring them back – keep on watching, protecting. When you ask God to use you and open your eye to get wisdom, understanding, and the spirit of discernment, these do happen. There's nothing that the Holy Spirit cannot give you when you ask prayerfully.

grandmother of three

On the other hand, one grandmother argues that wisdom is an illusion:

It's nice to believe that we have wisdom – it's a good illusion. There must be wonderful grandmothers who can tell stories. I would have loved to be one of them, but all I can do is churn out stories about the Greek Gods. I told my granddaughter the story of Paris and the Trojan War, but she didn't like it because they didn't get married and live happily ever after. I had to tell her I didn't know what happens to them in the end.

grandmother of five

And one suggests that it is not taken advantage of:

We do have the wisdom of our years, but the young people don't really allow it. All the younger mums these days, they want to do it their own way. Phone the NHS for any little thing and look it up on the internet, rather than listening to what we've got to offer. They don't even ask you. I don't feel very good about it. But my daughter knows how I brought them up and I notice some of the bits are there.

grandmother of one

Some suggest that wisdom begins earlier, with motherhood:

It takes wisdom when you've got children, you have to really think what is best for that child. A throwaway remark which might be cutting to an adult can be devastating to a child.

And you're always trying to set some kind of example. I might think it's okay to have five cigarettes a day, but I wouldn't say that in front of a child, because I'd want them not to do that. So you are monitoring yourself – there's a lot more responsibility when you're around children, because it's *all* example and repetition with kids.
grandmother of three

You need wisdom to understand the kids as well. It takes a lot to understand a child, to know where that child is coming from. It's hard work, bringing up a child.
grandmother of ten

Missing out on the pleasures
It has been seen that grandmothers, by and large, feel strongly that being a grandmother has added enormously to their lives. By extension, they also feel sorry for those cannot experience the pleasures – or choose not to:

People without grandchildren miss out on all these wonderful experiences and the love and the affection that you get from grandchildren. I have a friend who says, 'My daughter's had a baby, it's *her* job. I've done my bit, I've looked after my children, let her get on with it.' I'm stunned when people talk like that. They don't know what it is to have grandchildren and the love.

grandmother of two

Very few of my friends are actually grannies – only one, and she kicked against it for years: 'Oh, please don't have children – that's not for me – I'll be doing this, that, and the other'. I said to her, it won't be the same when it happens to you. And of course, as soon as it happens, you go into a big pile of mush – you just roll over and let them do whatever they want, because it's so lovely.

grandmother of one

If somebody says, 'My kid's having a kid soon and I don't want to be a grandmother,' I say, 'Wait. You might *think* you don't want to be a grandmother, but just wait.' I've got friends who've got no children. They really miss all of that. Watching the grandchildren grow up, going to their school plays, it's like having your own child again. All these things you do with them, it's like having it all twice.

grandmother of two

This may include grandfathers:

It's been a very loving experience. I try to be there. My ex-husband lives abroad and has never seen them. I find it strange. I think he's missing out terribly. It's a long time ago that he left, but I can't quite comprehend that you wouldn't want to know your grandchildren at all.

grandmother of two

And for those where there is no choice, there is particular sympathy:

> Women who don't have children miss out and it's a shame if there's no grandchildren. It kind of reconnects you again, when your child has a baby. I think it's fantastic to see your children have children. It's the moment when they stop being children. You're so proud of them going through it. My sister's got one child with severe mental health problems. I don't think he's going to find someone and have a child, and she is really heartbroken. She loves to hear about my grandchildren.
>
> ***grandmother of three***

But there is the occasional exception:

> Women who aren't grandmothers are lucky! They don't have to cook for them, don't have to do anything for them – just lucky they are. It is hard work to keep them on the straight and narrow.
>
> ***grandmother of ten***

End thoughts

We end as we began, with a few general thoughts from these very disparate grandmothers.

First, one might ask, what are grandmothers *for*? One woman calls attention to their importance in day-to-day child care:

> I read the New Scientist and there was some research, a few years ago, where they talked about humans being different from other mammals, because they're the only females that

don't remain fertile until they die. You have decades post-fertility – and what's that for?

I think it's a necessity because parents need the input, the back-up, to raise an infant. I do take the view that human society grew socially successful because it had that extra layer of input – in more ancient societies, the ancestors had a lot of importance.

Grandmothers need to be part of the fabric of family life, because every child needs lots of adults full-time to bring it up. A child's capacity to learn is limited only by the adults' capacity to teach them – and they just need as much input as is available. Yet it's a problem nowadays that everybody lives miles away from their family.

When I first lived here, everyone lived in walking distance to their work and to their mother-in-law. It was an intensely turned-inwards community and hostile to anybody who wasn't part of it, but it terms of having children, it worked like a charm. Modern life is not like that and losing that kind of support is a huge mistake. I hope that it's a late twentieth century blip and we'll come round to understanding that you need to live differently if you want to have children.

grandmother of two

Another notes how more grandmothers seem to be visible:

There's a lot of us grandmothers around, because there's more older people around.

250

Grandmothering has become more noticed and more 'done'. There are more grandmothers looking after their grandchildren, while the mothers and fathers work, than there used to be, because there's more grandparents available. We respect each other.

grandmother of two

And one comments on the impact of delayed parenthood:

People put far too much emphasis on having everything before you can have a child. It's absolute nonsense. You don't have to have a whole array of fancy gadgets and changing tables to have a child. Physically, and perhaps emotionally, people manage better when they have children in their twenties.

And the grandmothers also have more energy. In ten years, my youngest granddaughter will only be ten and I'll be in my 80s – and that's very different from having a ten year old when you're in your early 60s. It's the physical ability and the mental acuity to keep to grips with what's going on in the world.

grandmother of ten

Many ruminate on their actual involvement and what they have gained:

It's forced me to think about my relationship with those two little people, to make sure that I don't make many mistakes. It's a relationship that I value and I work at it. Maybe it's to do with age, but I think that they made me stop and think about *them* and it's very enriching for me.

Sometimes, they come and I feel tired afterwards, but it's a very positive thing. A friend once asked me – she's never married, has no children – 'What does it mean to you?' And I remember saying 'They are my life.' They just represent everything for me. I think it's remained like that, still.

grandmother of two

It's taught me to understand children better. My husband says he didn't enjoy our children, because he was out of the country travelling. I was busy running the home and doing things. I didn't enjoy children as I'm enjoying the grandchildren now. You can sit for hours, talk to them, play with them. I taught my grandchildren to ride a bike. We would spend hours together every Sunday afternoon.

grandmother of two

I've become more understanding. I've become less insistent that things have to be done a certain way. I was very disciplined with my girls, but I had to because I had four of them and their dad not around. With my grandson, I've become more relaxed, because it's not my responsibility, it's *her* responsibility.

grandmother of one

I feel privileged, blessed – very connected to the grandchildren. Grandmothering is merging with them sometimes and then standing back and looking at the bigger picture, which they can't see. Helping them to grow and reach out and understand – and delighting in that. It is lovely to be in intimate contact with a new being, seeing new things and having experiences for the very first time. It makes me feel new and puts me in touch with my own child self and my sense of wonder. It is life coming full circle.

grandmother of two

And some reiterate the joy of having created a large set of relationships:

I am just so proud. I only have to be looking at them, and I think, I can't believe that they're mine!' I feel like a bird puffing all his feathers out. Look at me, I'm so proud, look at what I've got. I've achieved. It's like a big achievement. Just the absolute joy of it all. I can't even put it into words.

grandmother of six

I like to think of myself as on the top of this great dynasty. It gives me a kick. It's absolutely fantastic to see another generation of something which you started yourself. It's a bit like empire-building. It's a great status. You've built another set somehow – and more people to love and to be yourself with. There's a kind of momentum where you know that when you die, they'll carry on somehow. I want it to be as big as possible – I'd be really upset if none of the grandchildren married and had children.

grandmother of three

One wishes she could slow time down:

I would probably say to anyone becoming a grandmother, just try to slow down and enjoy it more, slow the whole process down. You can't put people in a bubble, but I've often wanted to because this is just so wonderful. I've often wanted to say 'Oh, this is such a lovely time, let's just keep it like this, don't get any older.' But I had to stop myself saying that because the implication is that they'd die and that'd be it.

grandmother of one

And, after all these thoughts, one grandmother puts the case for just 'doing it':

I sometimes think, in today's world, people think too deeply about child-rearing. I tell my kids it's better just to get on with life and not think about it – just get on and live life. My identity as a grandmother is not something I think about. I just do it.

grandmother of eleven

About the author

Ann Richardson is a writer and researcher. She has written two previous books in a narrative style: *Wise Before their Time: People with AIDS and HIV talk about their lives* and *Life in a Hospice: reflections on caring for the dying.* She lives in London and is the grandmother of two boys.

Lightning Source UK Ltd.
Milton Keynes UK
UKOW02f1450121115

262573UK00002B/12/P